Healing with DMSO

Healing with DMSO

DMSO

the complete guide to safe and natural treatments for managing pain, inflammation, and other chronic ailments with dimethyl sulfoxide

Amandha Vollmer

ULYSSES PRESS

Published by:
ULYSSES PRESS
P. O. Box 3440
Berkeley, CA 94703
www.ulyssespress.com

ISBN: 978-1-64604-002-5
Library of Congress Control Number: 2019951340

Printed in the United States
10 9 8 7

Acquisitions editor: Casie Vogel
Managing editor: Claire Chun
Editor: Susan Lang
Proofreader: Renee Rutledge
Indexer: S4Carlisle
Front cover design: Hannah Rohrs
Cover art: © Cat arch angel gray/shutterstock.com

Contents

Introduction: DMSO, a Hidden Gem

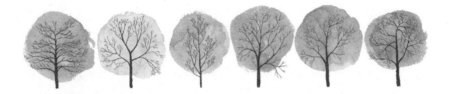

Who could imagine that a simple extract from trees could be one of the most powerful healers of all time? It may sound like a tall claim, but once you read about the science of DMSO (dimethyl sulfoxide) and the experiences people have had using it, I'm sure you will agree.

I first became aware of DMSO when learning about its use in sports medicine. An athlete incurs an injury and heads to the sidelines, where a medic immediately applies DMSO and assesses the situation; often the athlete is able to return to the game. I found it interesting, but I found so many remedies interesting. I thought, "Well, I'm not going into sports medicine so I probably won't need to use it," and pretty much forgot about it.

A decade later, after designing many natural skin care products and experimenting with hundreds of natural remedies, I was wandering around a health food store and noticed a bottle of DMSO on the shelf. I thought, "Hey, I haven't played around with this stuff, maybe I'll pick up a bottle," which I did. It sat on a shelf in my holistic medicine shop for many months, waiting for a customer to ask for it or for me to decide to use it in one of the creams or other unique products I formulate.

Soon after, a customer came in with a very strange rash on his forearms that appeared after a gardening session. The man said that it itched so badly, he was scratching his skin raw. It was worse at night, when he felt a crawling sensation. He had tried many creams and treatments, to no avail. I quickly realized that it must be a skin mite infection and instructed him to treat his skin with diatomaceous earth and 50 percent apple cider vinegar solution.

For some strange reason, the man kept touching me as he talked. When he left, I was so concerned about the mites spreading that I washed myself right away, but it was too late. Within a few days, when I experienced the same rash and itch, I used diatomaceous earth and apple cider vinegar on myself. While it seemed to help, I was still itchy and uncomfortable. I wondered if the DMSO (still sitting on my shelf) would speed my recovery. I grabbed the bottle containing a 90 percent solution of DMSO and applied the clear liquid to my right forearm. The warmth and burning were intense—and I loved the feeling that I had just applied something powerful! My skin became red and tingled. I applied it multiple times over a period of a few days and my skin became thick, almost leathery. (I would learn how to avoid that thickening, which I'll share later in this book.)

I needed to know what was going on. I dove almost obsessively into a study of DMSO. I read all of the published studies from the 1960s and all the early information, and what I read excited me to no end. There was a lot of information to absorb, but my ability to easily read studies coupled with my background in chemistry helped me to understand DMSO on a deep level in a short amount of time. DMSO can stop strokes and heart attacks? It deals with pain and is nonaddictive? It protects DNA from radiation damage with zero side effects? It increases nutrient absorption and utilization but also can protect the liver from drug damage? What?! I needed to tell everyone what I had learned. I had been producing videos on natural health for about a year to this point. So was born my video "All about DMSO, a Miracle Healer!," which has been extremely popular. My excitement and presentation were infectious. Since that time I have produced more videos on DMSO.

With my medical training, ability to research, knowledge of chemistry, awareness of the use of holistic medicine, and personal experience—along with designing and producing over a dozen successful DMSO product blends, helping others to use DMSO successfully and receiving their testimonials, and doing research for this book—I feel I am becoming a leading expert on the topic and that it chose me. Life has wonderful ways of bringing you flowers, and DMSO has been that kind of unexpected gift for me.

DMSO is a substance that every person should keep in the home, every parent should have in a first aid kit, and every doctor's office and hospital should have on hand. However, as you will learn, in North America it is a persecuted drug and I believe that its persecution has been fueled by misinformation, legal suppression, and medical dogma. This book sets out to dispel some of these myths and rumors, and to illuminate concrete facts about this incredible wood extract.

There are two main grades of purity (pharmaceutical and industrial) of this clear, colorless solvent, as well as a myriad of applications ranging from animal husbandry to sports medicine to organ transplantation. It can help with hair growth, cataract healing, and of course, all types of aches and pains. This book discusses specific applications for the medicinal use of DMSO and provides recipes you can whip up at home. But first, let's take a look at DMSO's history.

A Rocky History

A Russian doctor named Alexander M. Saytzeff discovered DMSO in 1866, yet no commercial application was identified until some nine decades later. In the 1950s, British scientists learned it could be used as a cryoprotective agent (protect against the harmful effects of freezing) to preserve bone marrow and blood cells. Frozen cells are irreparably damaged by ice crystallization. However, when DMSO is added to water and used as an antifreeze, it affects the thermodynamics of the freezing process in such a way that 85 percent of cells survive.[1] Cell viability and stabilization are essential in transplanting organs and preserving specimens for use in experiments. A substance that allows a tissue sample or organ to be frozen without damage and without altering the tissue in any negative way has huge value.

Scientists also found that DMSO was nontoxic to cells, which increased its versatility as a solvent. A solvent is simply a chemical that can dissolve a solute, making a solution. DMSO can dissolve anything that is either water or alcohol based as well as certain oil-based materials that are of a lighter molecular weight.

When Dr. Stanley Jacob at the Oregon Health and Science University Medical School discovered highly purified DMSO could penetrate skin and organ membranes without damaging them, he and his colleagues started looking more closely at its transdermal properties. They also found that DMSO is able to carry other substances of low molecular weight through the skin with it. However, we are getting a little ahead of the story …

Because of all its promising properties, Crown Zellerbach, one of the world's largest paper manufacturers in the 1950s, tasked one of its chemists, Robert Herschler, to find additional uses for DMSO. Because the company produced so much DMSO as a by-product of papermaking, it wanted to find a good use for the compound. As the proverb says, necessity is the mother of invention.

During his research, Herschler observed that antifungal agents and antibiotics were able to penetrate a plant's circulatory system when those materials were blended with DMSO. Although other chemicals like alcohol and gasoline did the same thing, DMSO was special. Herschler found that it did not damage or alter a plant's protective outer membrane. This begged the thought: If DMSO did not damage a plant's outer coating, perhaps the same would be true of DMSO applied to human skin.

Recognizing the potential medicinal applications, Herschler contacted his old friend Dr. Stanley Jacob, assistant professor of surgery at the University of Oregon. Dr. Jacob was specifically interested in cryobiology and was thrilled to be able to perform experimental research on a substance with such unique biological properties.

Oddly enough, DMSO got off to a bad start soon after initial research was completed. In 1963, newspapers in Oregon got hold of the patent information and sensationalized the properties of DMSO before it traversed the proper medical community channels. Because the word was already out, DMSO didn't have the chance to be introduced in scientific journals and backed up by studies, facts, and evidence. Rather, it came across as a hyped cure-all. Despite the substance having been tested on over 100,000 patients, with every study showing zero toxicity when used in the proper dosage, the FDA began to harass those involved with DMSO research. Dr. Jacob's laboratory and office were raided, patient files were copied without warrants, and Dr. Jacob himself was charged with producing insufficient and inconclusive evidence of DMSO's safety.[2]

So why the refusal to accept this research? DMSO was proven to be a safe, powerful, natural healing substance, yet it remained illegal. Why? It all came down to one negative study in which laboratory animals were given extremely high doses of DMSO via injection, which resulted in a clouding of the lens in the eye.[3] A negative side effect to be sure, but once the DMSO was halted, the lenses returned to normal in many of the animals. Nevertheless, the fate of the substance was sealed. On November 25, 1965, the FDA banned all use of DMSO.

There are a number of theories as to why the FDA did not wait to pass judgment on DMSO before more long-term studies could be conducted and analyzed. Some suggest it was due to the fact that they were still smarting from the recent thalidomide drug disaster, which maimed thousands of children and caused many miscarriages. This scandal led to tightened medical-testing regulations and greater limitations on medical conflicts of interest. The timing for DMSO being rediscovered wasn't ideal as the political climate was hesitant and overcautious, to a fault. Although thalidomide was never formally approved in the United States, a lawsuit filed in 2011 against the maker of the drug alleges that as many as 2.5 million doses of the drug were distributed by more than 1,200 doctors to more than 20,000 people, including pregnant women, in the United States.[4]

Others point to the fact that because no one drug company could obtain an exclusive patent (because DMSO is a natural compound), there is no possibility for a big financial return. Indeed, Stanley Jacob, considered the father of DMSO, stated that the controversies surrounding DMSO are, "bureaucratic and economic rather than scientific." In a *60 Minutes* interview in 1980, Dr. Jacob said that a large pharmaceutical executive told him, "I don't care if DMSO is the major drug of our century, and we all know it is, it isn't worth it to us."[5] He went on to say that although DMSO was competitive with other drugs, companies wanted nothing to do with it since they could not own and control it. The then-director of the Bureau of Drugs of the FDA, J. Richard Crout, said, "DMSO is a low toxicity and safe compound ... I think that it is a fact of life that drug companies are not going to invest in something unless they think there is some financial return."[6]

DMSO is the people's medicine. It is completely natural and very affordable. It is accessible to us because it is permitted for sale as a solvent and for use in veterinary medicine. It is FDA approved for horses as a topical medication. It is up to us to share this knowledge with others, to use DMSO in our lives and to demand medical access to it. One of the main purposes of this book is to spread DMSO awareness and let people know they have better solutions to their health problems than dangerous, suppressive, and sometimes addictive pharmaceutical drugs. Ensuring we stand up for our health freedom rights, in a world that is continually trying to reduce our health care choices, is an ever-important task for us all.

I invite you to journey with me as we explore the wisdom of the trees.

CHAPTER 1

The Chemistry of DMSO

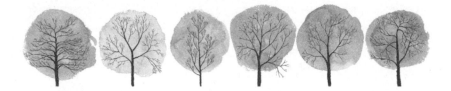

Dimethyl sulfoxide comes from tree lignin (an important component in plant cell walls) and is a by-product of the kraft method of pulp and paper production, also called the sulfate process. It also occurs naturally in the earth's sulfur cycle: DMS (dimethyl sulfide) is produced from marine phytoplankton in the oceans and then is oxidized into DMSO by the atmosphere. In fact, DMS is a cloud maker; its sulfur component turns into aerosols that water vapor surrounds, leading to cloud formation. Both DMS and DMSO compounds are vital to the marine sulfur cycle.[7] DMSO can also occur in certain foods, as we will explore later.

DMSO is a small molecule, only slightly larger than a water molecule, made up of carbon, hydrogen, sulfur, and oxygen atoms. The molecule contains a beautiful symmetry. It features one sulfur unit double bonded to an oxygen unit, flanked on either side by carbon and hydrogen methyl groups (CH3). Its molecular shape is reminiscent of water, which is known as the universal solvent. As a powerful solvent itself, DMSO is a close second to water. Because of its size, it is easily transported by the blood throughout the body. It mixes easily with both water and alcohol, dissolves both organic and inorganic substances, and readily moves through the skin's layers.

DMSO has a unique polarity, meaning that it has two faces, one that can attach to water-soluble molecules and one that can attach to oil-soluble molecules. Therefore, DMSO is amphiphilic—that is, both water loving (hydrophilic) and fat loving (lipophilic). Amphiphilic substances are also called surfactants and are commonly used in cleaning products. When you think about it, it really does make sense that these substances are perfect for cleaning dishes, counters, and even your body!

In water, DMSO's polarity can alter the spaces between its own molecules, a phenomenon called conformation. The order and spacing of those molecules then determine what kind of action DMSO can perform. Form is function. For example, when the molecules' configuration is malleable, DMSO can interact with proteins and move through them. This malleable configuration is why DMSO can travel with ease through the skin's surface. This is also one of the main reasons for its analgesic (pain-killing) properties. DMSO in water affects nerve membranes and reduces their sensitivity, leading to a reduction of pain signals. You can see why DMSO makes such a great pain reliever. This is something we will discuss in greater depth in later chapters.

DMSO's sulfur-oxygen bond is also very polar, which results in something called dipole attraction.[8] Think of it as a plus and a minus on either end of a stick. The two ends are attracted to each other and also to other plus and minus energy, which drives their complex folding dance. The stick bends to make ends meet, but also to attach to the ends of other sticks. This dipole interaction is critical for a very important effect in nature called protein folding. To perform their biological function, protein molecules need to fold into a distinct three-dimensional shape. Unfolded proteins are generally inactive but can sometimes be harmful. The way in which a protein folds is dependent on dipole-dipole interactions (the ends of the stick), and DMSO's dipole interaction can explain many of its biological actions on living organisms.

Let's go back to the fact that DMSO can easily move through the membranes of plants and the skin of people and animals. DMSO exchanges sites with bound water molecules. Imagine dancers grabbing hands in an alternating fashion moving through a line. One after the other, they make their way down the line, all the while exchanging handshakes with new partners. This is how DMSO moves through tissue, exchanging hands with water.

In 2017, scientists at the University of Texas ran a study on the hydrogen bonds that form between DMSO and water. The study found that at low concentrations, DMSO forms two hydrogen bonds with water; at medium concentrations, it forms only one hydrogen bond with water; at very high concentrations, it ignores water and clumps with other DMSO molecules.[9] These results provide valuable insight on proper dosing for a wide range of health and industry applications. The dosage always matters in medicine, but with DMSO's unique chemistry, it's even more important to understand. We will talk about dosing later on in this book.

Another interesting component of DMSO's chemistry is its high freezing point and melting point. A melting point is the temperature at which a solid changes to the liquid state, whereas freezing point is the point at which a liquid changes to a solid. These temperatures should be close to identical. Fascinatingly, in its pure state, DMSO readily freezes at 65.4°F; its melting point is specifically 65.12°F. Often, people find that their DMSO has solidified overnight during winter, even in the warmth of the house. There is no cause for concern, just a little time at a temperature above 65.4°F and DMSO returns to its liquid state. You don't have to worry that the substance will expand and break its container the way that water can, because water expands at a rate 230 times higher than DMSO when it moves from a liquid to a solid state. I recommend storing pure (99.995 percent) DMSO in glass, although it is inert or nonreactive in certain plastics like PETE (polyethylene terephthalate). However, if you're unsure of what your plastic containers are made of, it's better to be safe than sorry and go with glass.

DMSO as a Transdermal Agent

The word "transdermal" means to cross the skin, so anything that has transdermal qualities is able to pass through the skin and into the tissues below and the bloodstream. DMSO has transdermal properties and can move through the skin in three fascinating ways.

One, it can switch places with water molecules.

Two, it can cause both hydrophobic (meaning it repels water) and hydrophilic (meaning it mixes with water) responses in the skin's pores, weakening the electro-mechanical forces and allowing the DMSO and whatever it is carrying to pass through.

Three, at higher concentrations, DMSO can cause the fat molecules in our cell membranes (called ceramides), to transition from a dense gel state to liquid crystalline.[10,11] In this liquid crystalline state, the ceramides show liquid properties while also having molecules that are arranged in a crystal-like manner. DMSO stimulates this shift in state, allowing the DMSO and whatever it is carrying to pass through the ceramides and deeper into our tissue below the skin. Clearly the concentration of DMSO applied to the skin will affect the method in which it will traverse the skin's surface. The repeated ceramide changes of state are what caused the reddening and thickening of my skin when I first experimented with it. Diluting it further with water would have allowed the dipolar movement through my skin to occur, causing less skin changes.

Sulfa, Sulfate, Sulfites, and Sulfur

Fun fact: It is actually not possible to be allergic to elemental sulfur. It is a vital element to life on Earth and has no protein content that can cause an allergic reaction. When people say they are "allergic" to sulfur, what they really mean is that they are allergic to sulfur-containing drugs, foods, or proteins. It is important to understand that the chemistry of pure elemental sulfur is different from that of sulfur-containing chemicals.

Sulfur-containing drugs, such as sulfa antibiotics (sulfonamides) or preservatives known as sulfites, which are used in wines, dried fruit, and other foods, can cause a histamine reaction. This means that an allergic reaction has occurred in which histamines are released in the body, triggering symptoms like inflammation. Sulfates are used in shampoos and body washes to increase foaming, and some people are very sensitive to them. The two most common sulfates are sodium lauryl sulfate (SLS) and sodium laureth sulfate (SLES). You've probably seen a lot of shampoos and conditioners with the words "sulfate free" on their packaging. It's becoming more and more common nowadays, which is great for our hair and scalps, reducing the chemical load in our bodies.

Sometimes people are sensitive to foods that have a high sulfur content, such as garlic, onions, broccoli, and cauliflower. Often, there are some other issues going on with these individuals as well. They may have nutritional deficiencies, especially a deficiency in the trace mineral molybdenum, which enzymes need to oxidize sulfur compounds such as sulfites to sulfates. These individuals also tend to have an unbalanced gut microbiome (which is composed of the bacteria in the intestines). Generally, individuals with these problems can also have genetic mutations in genes like MTHFR or COMT and should avoid synthetic folic acid (found in a variety of supplements), take methylfolate and methylcobalamin (B12) supplements, and I also suggest using the supplement TMG or DMG (trimethylglycine or dimethylglycine) in order to give important methyl groups to the body. Methyl groups tag DNA, proteins, and amino acids to ensure proper folding and support many other key processes in the body.

Most individuals with allergies to sulfa drugs, sulfites, or foods high in sulfur content do not experience problems taking DMSO, because apart from its sulfur component, DMSO bears no relation to these substances.[12] The same goes for other sulfur-containing substances: MSM, alpha-lipoic acid, allicin (the main active ingredient in garlic), glucosamine sulfate (and its natural polymer chondroitin), SAMe (S-adenosylmethionine), and several valuable antioxidants such as glutathione and N-acetylcysteine (NAC).

DMSO Grade

Understanding that there are different grades of DMSO is important, especially if you are planning on using it for your health. There are two main grades, pharmaceutical and industrial. The industrial grade must come with a warning that it is not intended for human use. It is wise to contact the manufacturer if you are unsure of a product's purity. The only grade that should be used in humans or animals is pharmaceutical grade, or 99.995 percent purity. To achieve this percentage, activated charcoal is run through the DMSO at the end of filtering to ensure no other impurities are present.

In its industrial grade, DMSO has many applications. In addition to its use as a less toxic additive to paint-stripping formulations, it is used in the formation of polymers as a reactive solvent, and in agriculture for ingredient synthesis (for example, in making antifungals for plants). It is also used in cleaning applications because it is an environmentally safe alternative to toxic chemicals and acts in a similar way to detergents.

Despite its history with the FDA, pharmaceutical-grade DMSO is certainly not underused, although its application is limited. It is now incorporated into a number of regulated products for health care and drug delivery applications (see Chapter 8), especially as an excipient (a substance that is inactive and is used as a bulking agent, a diluting agent, or as a vehicle for an active drug). DMSO stabilizes formulated products and can dissolve many difficult or "stubborn" materials. Plus, it can absorb alcohols, fats, minerals, vitamins, amino acids, and carbohydrates without damaging them.[13] All of these properties make it very useful in medical and pharmaceutical situations.

Remember the history of DMSO? Scientists found that it could protect human cells and tissues from being damaged when frozen. This is why pharmaceutical-grade DMSO is used during organ transplants, during which the organs are put on ice. The DMSO helps to preserve the organ's cells against freezing while on ice. DMSO when added to water depresses its freezing point significantly. In some cases, priming the body with DMSO helps prevent many common drug side effects and reduces post-surgical complications, for example, radiation damage.[14] In other cases, DMSO can enhance a drug or treatment.

I could fill many books with information about the combination of DMSO with various drugs or natural substances. DMSO can be used to open up the tissues of the skin or inside the body to receive nutrients, botanicals, homeopathics, or any other medicine. Blending with other medicines allows DMSO to carry those substances into the bloodstream and past the blood–brain barrier. This provides the body with greater access to any substance that DMSO attaches to and transports. If you can imagine all the possible DMSO combinations, it's a massive topic! My focus here is on the most important remedies for use in the home. DMSO partners well with so many remedies that the future of DMSO can be a very bright one, if we create it.

Other Forms of DMSO

Besides its pharmaceutical and industrial uses, DMSO is naturally found in many of the common foods we eat and drink, like tea, coffee, wine, asparagus, clams, tomatoes, milk, and cooked corn.[15] It has been isolated in spearmint oil, nonfat dried milk, barley malt, and natural waters. It is the end product of algal metabolism (the results of algae taking up and converting nutrients into other materials). It is also excreted in small amounts in our urine and is found in the urine of other mammals. This means that even during pregnancy and breastfeeding, small amounts of DMSO exposure to the fetus or child is recognizable.

Conclusion

Now that you are more familiar with DMSO, its unique chemistry, its wide application, and its interesting history, let's discuss how to use it safely and properly. I am also going to teach you some important aspects of the human body so that the suggested applications make more sense. There is nothing to fear with DMSO. So many people approach me, afraid they'll use it incorrectly or afraid to use it at all, and I tell them how safe it actually is. Knowledge is power and applied wisdom is always more guided than guesswork. Once you understand the dos and don'ts of DMSO, you will feel confidence in using it for all kinds of applications. It will become a go-to for a wide variety of ailments.

CHAPTER 2

DMSO's Major Actions

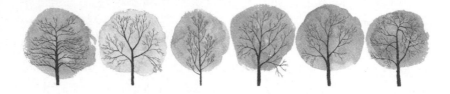

The Healing Crisis

Even though DMSO has been labeled as a drug, it is actually a natural healing compound, one found in nature—in both plants and foods. Unlike synthetic compounds, which can suppress symptoms (instead of heal symptoms) or overwhelm the body, the majority of natural substances stimulate and encourage the body's innate healing mechanisms. The key to all medicines, whether synthetic or naturally occurring, is proper dosage and application.

We all know that any substance, even everyday household drugs like ibuprofen or acetaminophen, can be misused or overdosed upon. Depending on their health, different people can show hypersensitivities or no response at all to the same dosage. This is because our bodies are unique. The same is true when using DMSO. People whose bodies have accumulated all sorts of environmental debris, food wastes, and heavy metals, or who are not exercising, eating well, or managing their stress properly are more likely to have a "reaction" when they first begin using DMSO. During my 10-plus years of educating people about their health, I see this response again and again. Also known as a healing crisis, this "reaction" or detoxification process occurs when the body is stimulated into healing, but the debris must be cleared out for healing to occur.

Many of my clients have congested kidneys and livers, two of the primary routes of waste filtration and elimination. When they do use DMSO, or almost any natural healing approach, they may experience detoxification symptoms or a pathogenic die-off reaction (also called a Herxheimer reaction). The symptoms vary, but the most common are headaches, nausea, fatigue, bowel changes, skin rashes, mood changes, and bloating. In extreme but rare cases, I see true histamine-type reactions, itching, swelling or hives, blood pressure and heart rate changes, and, even more rarely, anaphylactic reactions. Such an intense reaction occurs only because the DMSO is mixing with something else in the body and this mixture is what the body is reacting to. You cannot be allergic to the simple components of DMSO, which are carbon, hydrogen, oxygen, and sulfur, or else you'd be allergic to your own body. As we discussed, DMSO contains no complex protein for the body to react to. Detox symptoms are what the body creates while it is healing. As a holistic practitioner, I want to help the body to do what it desires in a proper manner without complications, providing resolution. This is a central principle of holistic healing.

Drug or Nature's Medicine?

No synthetic drug can give the body its fundamental building blocks (called biochemicals) that run all our metabolic systems, rebuild cells and tissues, and remove waste materials. In fact, most synthetic drugs can cause nutritional deficiencies. For example, look at the popular statin drugs, which are designed to reduce cholesterol. A 1998 study found that statin drugs cause deficiencies in coenzyme Q10, or CoQ10, which is vital for heart function.[16, 17] CoQ10 is also called "ubiquinone" because it is ubiquitous in animals and most bacteria. An important antioxidant, it is vital for energy production in cells and specifically heart muscle cells. However, the majority of individuals who tell me they are taking a statin drug are not taking a CoQ10 supplement even though Dr. Julian Whitaker, MD, filed a petition in 2002 urging the FDA to include CoQ10 on all statin drug labeling.[18] Moreover, we have known statins deplete CoQ10 since at least 1990.[19]

Nutritional deficiencies are just one of the many side effects that can be caused by synthetic drug use. Natural healing substances do not generally cause such high levels of nutritional deficiencies, as they work with the body and contain materials the body needs. DMSO, for example, offers the body methyl groups (consisting of carbon and hydrogen, basic building blocks of life), elemental sulfur, and oxygen.

Other side effects are caused by bodily systems that can no longer operate properly because the drug is overriding a signal to either increase or decrease the production of a certain biochemical end product. Generally, when more of an end product is made, the signal calls for reduced levels. When that end product starts to run thin, the signal calls for increased production once again. This control allows the body to keep everything in balance. But when a drug overrides the signal, that signal can't do its job, and end product levels can go haywire. This can lead to imbalances like memory problems, muscle pain, and other neurological problems.[20]

DMSO has never been shown to induce symptoms even marginally close to what certain synthetic drugs can cause, yet these drugs, like statins, continue to be prescribed.[21] I can give examples of this trend again and again with blood pressure medication, acetaminophen, corticosteroids, antibiotics, and the list goes on, with many more drugs coming down the pike. For me, it's frustrating that a safe, effective, easy-to-administer, affordable substance like DMSO has not been fully brought to the public's awareness.

DMSO and Pharmaceutical Drug Use

Using DMSO while on any drug is risky, as the combined action in addition to the uniqueness of each individual can be unpredictable. Although DMSO is safe to use in the correct dosage and on its own, it can act as a catalyst to allow drugs easier and greater access into the body. I do not recommend using DMSO if you are on prescription medication, and you should consult with your doctor or pharmacist before making any changes to your medication regimen.

There is only one case of a DMSO-related human death on record. In the 1960s in Ireland, a woman who had been on a course of antibiotics was also on anti-anxiety medication and had an anaphylactic reaction to DMSO, but still continued to take it despite her negative reaction.[22] Her resulting death was an extremely unfortunate and preventable tragedy; her histamine reaction should have been a clear signal to stop her dosage.

Although pairing DMSO with any pharmaceutical should generally be avoided and if done, should be done with only the utmost caution, DMSO should absolutely not be taken with diuretic drugs. This is because DMSO is also a diuretic, and pairing two diuretics is dangerous. Because DMSO has an affinity for water, any medication that alters kidney function should not be used in conjunction with DMSO.

Mostly what studies have shown, however, is that DMSO tends to take on a protective role in the presence of most drugs. It is true that in the pharmaceutical industry, DMSO is used to assist active drugs as it is an inactive substance. It is also used to bulk up or dilute certain drugs. In this way, DMSO can also be used in combination with certain drugs to assist their action and reduce the amount of drug required. I have devoted Chapter 5 to DMSO combinations that can be used to enhance other therapies and natural remedies.

DMSO and Other Products of Nature

As we learned earlier, DMSO is absorbed rapidly through the skin. Because the skin has both water- and oil-soluble barriers, DMSO's bipolar nature allows it to traverse those layers quickly. That being said, the absorption rate depends on the individual, and people with fair skin tend to show greater sensitivity, redness, and itching when DMSO passes through the barriers.

DMSO paves the way for bigger molecules, such as essential oils, to pass through by "making inner skin layers and underlying tissue reversibly accessible, sometimes even on nanoscale level."[23] What this means is that DMSO makes the skin accessible for materials to pass through it, and also out from within (i.e., to push out or expel toxins). The nanomolecular scale is a very small size of particle, and because DMSO assists nanoparticles through the cells, it is used in research to transfer very tiny-sized DNA particles into cells.[24] Given DMSO's special traits, combining it with natural substances like vitamins, minerals, botanicals, and even homeopathics open up a whole new level of therapeutic value than DMSO on its own. In my opinion, the sky's the limit for creating useful DMSO combinations to heal all sorts of health conditions.

DMSO's Activities

DMSO has very specific and powerful actions in humans, animals, and plants, some of which were discussed earlier. Here's a summary list of a number of those actions. I will go more fully into some of these following the list:[25]

- Has antimicrobial properties

- Is a muscle relaxant

- Increases production of white cells and macrophages, important cells for the immune system

- Increases cell membrane permeability, allowing for removal of toxins

- Is radioprotective, reducing the mutagenic and lethal effects of x-rays

- Inhibits cholinesterase enzyme from breaking down acetylcholine, an important neurotransmitter

- Is an excellent heavy metal detoxifier, binding to aluminum, mercury, cadmium, arsenic, and nickel and eliminating them through urination and sweating

- Is an effective pain killer, blocking nerves conducting pain signals

- Exhibits cryoprotective properties. Helps preserve stem cells, bone marrow cells, and organs (protecting against injury from freezing during organ transportation) and protects against damage during interstitial cystitis and cancer radiation therapy (both uses FDA approved)

- Is a bacteriostatic agent, meaning it inhibits the growth of bacteria

- Acts as a diuretic

- Reduces inflammation and swelling by affecting inflammatory chemicals
- Improves blood supply to injured areas by dilating blood vessels and reducing blood viscosity
- Increases delivery of oxygen to the cells
- Is a potent free radical scavenger, transporting these substances through excretory organs
- Is transdermal, easily penetrating the skin and blood–brain barrier, and enters the bloodstream
- Protects the cells from mechanical damage more rapidly than pharmaceutical drugs
- Has a calming effect on the central nervous system
- Acts as a carrier for all other drugs and supplements and increases their effects; for example, chemotherapy, corticosteroids, antibiotics, and insulin show less undesirable effects and can be used in much smaller quantities
- Has antinociceptive properties, meaning that it reduces the sensitivity to any dangerous or harmful stimuli
- Is nontoxic and has an unquestionably safe therapy profile

Works as an Anti-inflammatory Agent

Inflammation is a response to tissue injury. Consequences of inflammation under the skin are redness, heat, swelling, pain, and reduced function. In general, inflammation is just plain uncomfortable! Luckily, DMSO is a remarkable anti-inflammatory agent, helping to remove specific biological markers such as cytokines, histamine, bradykinin, prostaglandins, and leukotrienes, and speeding tissue repair. Scientists first discovered the anti-inflammatory action of DMSO when conducting experiments.[26, 27] They theorized that this beneficial mechanism might be due to the effect of DMSO on prostaglandin (fat molecules found in almost all human tissue) pathways, which are key players in the inflammatory response. These fat molecules, which operate like a hormone, are derived from arachidonic acid, an omega-6 fatty acid that promotes skeletal muscle tissue repair and is also found abundantly in the brain. However, too much arachidonic acid can lead to tissue damage and inflammation, as well as further aggravate symptoms. People whose diets are high in animal fat show increased production of arachidonic acid, which, in excess or in imbalance with omega-3, -9, or -12, can lead to chronic inflammation and other health issues.

So how does DMSO help with inflammatory responses? As I said above, DMSO has a substantial effect on prostaglandin pathways.[28] First, it helps to widen arteries (vasodilation) and prevents them from constricting (vasoconstriction), allowing for better blood flow. Bringing improved blood flow to an injured region is always necessary for healing, as the blood moves wastes away and brings in the mediators of healing.

In addition, DMSO increases the production of a molecule called cAMP, important in the formation of platelets.[29] Platelets are needed for forming blood clots to stop bleeding, but it's important that these platelets don't improperly clump into clots that cause stroke or brain injury. This is where DMSO can be beneficial, as it encourages the making of platelets but not their clumping. It also reduces the production of a molecule called thromboxane, which causes blood vessels to constrict. When DMSO reduces this molecule, blood vessels open (or dilate) more, allowing for greater blood to flow to an area of the body. With more blood flow comes more nutrient delivery, waste removal, cell-to-cell communication, and greater healing. So DMSO affects three pathways (vasodilation, vasoconstriction, and platelet separation) related to clot formation and encouraging blood flow. From just these actions, we can see how powerful and important DMSO is in so many disease situations.

If that weren't enough, DMSO is a natural nonsteroidal anti-inflammatory drug (NSAID). This means DMSO acts much like aspirin: Both work by blocking prostaglandins and controlling on-off switches in certain cells that regulate inflammation and pain.[30, 31, 32] DMSO is even better at this than aspirin as it also stops or slows the conduction of nerve fibers.[33] These nerve fibers are sensory nerves that transmit pain signals to the brain.[34] They are nonmyelating, meaning they are smaller fibers of the central nervous system and do not have a cover, or myelin sheath, on them. Whereas aspirin and other NSAIDs are considered toxic to the stomach, causing ulcers and irritation, and can lead to eye damage (macular degeneration) and cartilage damage, DMSO does not have these actions. DMSO can even help with musculoskeletal pain disorders when consistently and correctly applied over time.

Antioxidant or Pro-oxidant?

DMSO is such a fascinating substance, with the ability both to remove reactive oxygen species (ROS), which can harm the body as free radicals, and to oxidize certain tissues that are in need of destruction (for example, cancer cells). We must, therefore, understand how DMSO dosages and blends can affect the chemical action on the body and use the appropriate knowledge to tackle the specific health situation with effectiveness.

DMSO can act as a mild or potent antioxidant or pro-oxidant, depending on the percentage used, the pH of the tissue that absorbs DMSO, the materials it interacts with, and the user's health. Antioxidant and pro-oxidant activity must be balanced by the body to avoid producing too much oxidative stress. However, what is interesting is that both are needed for various health reasons. Pro-oxidants kill bacteria and fungus via the white blood cells, and during times of growth or injury, remove damaged tissue and wastes. Antioxidants are needed to prevent heart disease, cancers, immune dysfunction, and metabolic disorders.[35] A negative effect of an antioxidant is thus called a pro-oxidant effect.[36] Pro-oxidation targets damaged cells and triggers programmed cell death, which is sometimes desired but sometimes inappropriate. For example, a study of heel pressure ulcers showed that a 5 percent DMSO application produced a worse outcome than the controls.[37] In that study, DMSO acted as a pro-oxidant, donating its oxygen molecule into the biochemical reaction. In another important study for industrial production of furans, results showed that DMSO could be used to oxidize copper.[38] Furans are generally known as toxic by-products; however, they are also used as starting materials in various industries. DMSO generally only can act as a mild pro-oxidant; however, in high enough dosages it has the reputation of being a king of antioxidant activity. DMSO takes the place of water inside a living cell so it is able to destroy intracellular free radicals. No other antioxidant can do that.[39] It directly reduces the production of hydroxyl free radicals, as shown in a study done on various tissue samples.[40] A study of lung injuries found that 0.02 percent DMSO (injectable) was a very powerful antioxidant.[41] In the case of DMSO as an oxidant, it is always wise to take certain vitamins and minerals to neutralize any free radicals that the DMSO may produce. Some good ones that I recommend are vitamins A, E, C, B1, and B6 as well as zinc and selenium. In this day and age, I generally suggest that everyone take a B-complex vitamin in the morning after breakfast, for energy and detoxification.

Crosses the Blood–Brain Barrier

A 1982 study conducted on mice used an injection of 10 to 15 percent DMSO and an enzymatic tracer (which is used as a biological marker) that is usually unable to cross the blood–brain barrier.

However, it was later found in the brains of the test subjects, which meant the DMSO allowed the tracer to cross the barrier.[42] That was powerful evidence that DMSO crosses the blood–brain barrier and allows other molecules entrance into the brain. This action has huge implications for treating head injury, brain cancer, cerebral stroke, and other brain diseases. The fact that DMSO allows chemotherapy agents access to the brain should persuade doctors in this field to employ it more widely, but DMSO is not generally used, again highlighting how suppressed the knowledge of it still is. We will discuss this further in later sections of this book.

Protects Against Radiation Damage and Promotes DNA Repair

Of all DMSO's traits, these are the ones I personally find most fascinating. For a substance to prevent the damaging effects of ionizing radiation (which carries enough energy to break molecular bonds and add ions to atoms, much more energy than non-ionizing radiation) on DNA is simply amazing. We've all learned in school that radiation is dangerous. Radiation produces free radicals, sometimes called inflammatory molecules, which damage the cells that make our organs, glands, muscles, and bones. Ionizing radiation causes the cells to age more quickly and to become distorted or mutated, resulting in birth defects, anemia, cancers such as leukemia, and other diseases.

Before we get into how DMSO can promote DNA repair after radiation damage, let's have a quick refresher on DNA itself. You probably remember from middle school science class that DNA consists of double-stranded helices that carry the blueprints for our genetic structure. Their proper function is vital to life. In our cells, DNA is transcribed into messenger RNA. The RNA carries the information to the ribosomes inside the cell, which are like mini factories that create a chain of amino acids in a process called translation. These chains fold into proteins that are essential to every system in the body.

Strands of DNA can and do break—in fact, thousands of them daily—but the body works to repair the damage. These breaks can occur from mechanical stress on the cell, ionizing radiation, and chemical damage, such as free radical damage caused by ROS. If the DNA is damaged, genetic information important for making new cells may be lost. Fortunately, the body has a number of mechanisms available to repair DNA.

Both single- and double-strand breaks can occur in the DNA double helix. DMSO has been shown to accelerate DNA strand break repair and to prevent the initial damage from ionizing radiation.[43] DMSO helps prevent radiation damage by increasing the levels of glutathione (GSH). If the levels of the active form of GSH in the body drop to lower than 70 percent, cellular dysfunction occurs, leading to disease. GSH ensures that the ROS created by radiation are unable to damage the cell.

Applying DMSO to the body or taking it internally before undergoing any procedure involving radiation can be a wise decision for preventing DNA damage and the damaging effects of free radicals.[44] As well, the radioprotective effects can prevent ulcers caused by radiation therapy used in conventional cancer therapy from forming.

DMSO also assists after radiation exposure. I maintain the viewpoint that, when it comes to radiation exposure, the sooner one can apply DMSO, the better. For minor exposures, like head CT or a mammogram, I prescribe the following:

Combine 1 teaspoon of pure 99.995 percent DMSO in 5 ounces of distilled water or juice. Drink this mixture daily for seven days straight.

For higher radiation exposures, like a full-body CT, a larger dose of DMSO can be used. I recommend the following:

Cover the body with 80 percent DMSO as soon as possible. Dilute 1 ounce of pure DMSO into 1 ounce of distilled water or juice. Drink this 2-ounce mixture twice a day. The combination of these two treatments could relieve radiation side effects and help heal damaged DNA. However, prevention using DMSO is far more effective than trying to repair the damage afterward.

Imagine if those who work in nuclear power plants, radiation technicians, flight crews, or those in iron and uranium mining were educated on DMSO, if it could be used as part of a workplace health and safety strategy to prevent radiation damage. This is an achievable goal that I hope someone undertakes in these industries.

Restrains Bacterial Growth

DMSO has been shown to be bacteriostatic, meaning it restrains bacterial growth, which allows the immune system to deal with the situation properly. In one study a 20 percent DMSO concentration was found to control the growth of the bacteria E. coli, Staphylococcus aureus, and Pseudomonas.[45] Studies have also found DMSO to have antifungal and antiparasitic properties.[46]

Antibiotic-resistant bacteria in hospital settings are an ever-growing problem, increasing morbidity, hospital stays, and more expensive treatments.[47] Many antibiotics attack bacteria by inactivating a protein essential to them. There are two ways that bacteria become resistant to the attacks. One is through genetic change, by stimulating the protein to mutate so the antibiotic no longer recognizes it; the other is by increasing the production of that protein so there is more of it. Adding DMSO to drug-resistant antibiotics allows for reversion to antibiotic sensitivity, so the drug once again is effective against the bacteria.[48]

Increases Vasodilation

One of the important properties of DMSO is its exothermic reactivity, meaning it produces heat when it comes into contact with other substances, particularly water. Not all exothermic reactions are considered therapeutic, but DMSO's reactivity may be significant.[49] A study found that topical application of DMSO increased skin temperature, as well as the temperature of the layers of tissue beneath the skin.[50] The researchers deduced that this was a heat-liberating reaction by cells and tissues, and could signify vasodilation. So too, the redness that we generally see with topical application of DMSO is an indicator of vasodilation.

So what is vasodilation and why is it so important? As mentioned, vasodilation is the widening (a.k.a. dilation) of blood vessels. This happens naturally when you exercise, when you are in a hot environment, and even when you drink alcohol. Vasodilation is important because it can lower blood pressure while increasing blood flow to different parts of your body.

With such promising properties, it shouldn't come as a surprise that DMSO can be used as a powerful stroke preventive treatment, as well as first aid in an emergency. Indeed, this particular action of DMSO is what makes it so well loved in the treatment of both headaches and strokes. Many cardiac problems stem from a lack of oxygen delivery to tissues, and vasodilation and oxygen delivery go hand in hand. This can be due to a low oxygen level (hypoxia) or no oxygen delivery at all (anoxia). There are different types of strokes. An ischemic stroke is caused by low blood supply or oxygen delivery; a hemorrhagic stroke is caused by a bleed-out. In the case of ischemic stroke, DMSO should be used as first aid and given in a high dose by injection or orally.

It has been proposed that DMSO may reduce oxygen use by an inhibiting effect on mitochondria, little organs inside the cell that make energy in the form of adenosine triphosphate (ATP).[51] In one experiment, an increase in glycolysis, or cellular respiration, compensated for energy loss due to the slowing down of oxidative activity after brain tissue was perfused with DMSO.[52] The body starts to burn more glucose to make more energy and encourage more oxygen in the bloodstream. So the DMSO makes the body think it doesn't have enough oxygen and the body gets moving to give it more!

Repairs Wounds and Ulcers

DMSO is an excellent wound healer. It reduces ROS, a cause of cell destruction leading to dead tissue (necrosis) and a problem in ulcer creation. For example, a large amount of ROS is present in bed sores, also called pressure ulcers. Using DMSO early on, before ulcers are fully formed, has been shown to halt their production entirely, and applying DMSO to existing bed sores speeds healing.[53] Oftentimes the issue with bed sores is lack of blood flow to an area of damage, either on the outside of the body or the inside. DMSO repairs the tissue, allows blood to move to an area of damage, and introduces other substances paired with it to accelerate tissue repair. In the situation of bed sores, DMSO promotes blood transport into the local blood vessels to stimulate the healing process.

Ulcers and wounds are specific tissue injuries, and DMSO can be used wherever we see tissue injury.[54] This type of injury usually begins because of a lack of blood flow due to poor nutrition, poisoning, inflammation, or a physical injury like an accident. DMSO has found success in treating scleroderma, allergic eczema, contact dermatitis, rheumatoid arthritis, and pain syndromes, all of which feature tissue damage from long-standing inflammation.[55]

CHAPTER 3

DMSO Precautions

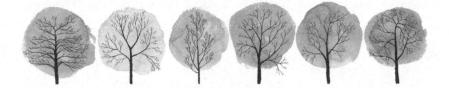

Knowledge is power. The proper use of DMSO will help to ensure a more successful outcome. While the likelihood of DMSO causing harm is minuscule, we must always act with wisdom and caution when using any type of medicine. I have included as much detail as I can into this section, so you feel well-educated and therefore more comfortable with your use of DMSO.

Skin Irritation

The most common issue with DMSO that I hear about is the temporary warmth, redness, peeling, itching, swelling, or burning it can cause to the skin. As far as side effects go, most of these are quite minor. To diminish them, you can reduce the percentage of DMSO you use. When it comes to the suggested percentages in this book, always adjust them for your own unique skin type and body depending on the reactions you see. One thing to keep in mind is that DMSO can also react with the dyes in tattoos, so it must not be applied on a tattoo site. It can take the dyes deeper into the body, which is not desired, as the majority of tattoo inks are toxic.

A natural partner for DMSO is the succulent plant aloe vera. You've probably seen aloe vera used for sunburns, and it is also known for its anti-inflammatory properties. Its cooling effect balances out the heat and redness that DMSO can cause. Often this combination is sold as a DMSO gel containing a ratio of 90 percent DMSO to 10 percent preservative-free aloe vera gel juice. Although some people can tolerate 90 percent DMSO, I find that this dilution is not necessarily ideal. In general, between 40 and 80 percent DMSO is best for topical applications. The lower end of that range is advisable for animals or on sensitive skin like the face, while the higher end of the range is suitable for thicker or tougher skin, like on the soles of the feet.

We've learned that DMSO increases blood flow to the skin (vasodilation), which explains the redness that occurs when using the substance at the proper dosage. The redness soon fades afterwards, generally within anywhere from 5 to 20 minutes. Keep in mind that I do not generally recommend using DMSO in dilutions higher than 80 percent repeatedly on the skin. Higher percentages can cause a different kind of redness due to swelling and thickening of the skin. This unwanted side effect will calm, and the skin will return to normal a few days after the usage of high-percentage DMSO is stopped.

Using 99.995% strength DMSO on the skin does have its place, and from time to time I do apply it in this manner, especially in the treatment of small wounds, pimples, or scar tissue. I have had much feedback about using it full strength and many people use it this way with great effectiveness. However, to keep the skin from peeling and thickening, I advise against applying full-strength DMSO repeatedly on the same patch of skin.

Individual sensitivity to DMSO can vary considerably. I have customers and clients tell me that higher percentages of DMSO caused them no irritation, while others say they had a very hard time with tingling, burning, and itching. I have found that hormones can dictate sensitivity. The higher the estrogen levels, the more sensitive the individual. For example, women may notice different sensitivities at different times of their menstrual cycle. If you find that a 70 percent solution is too irritating for you, then decrease it by 10 percent and test it, and keep testing until you find a percentage you can tolerate. A 40 percent solution is the lowest you should go for topical use. However, keep in mind that in cases of extremely sensitive skin, a percentage lower than 40 might be necessary.

With any new substance, it is always wise to apply a small amount as a test patch, usually on the inside of the wrist. This will give you feedback on how sensitive you are to DMSO and to the percentage you are using. Any redness, itching, tingling, or burning sensation should fade after about 10 minutes or so, although redness can take up to 20 minutes to fade completely. This is the average time it takes for DMSO to cross the skin barrier. I have not read about or heard of anyone who experienced a long-term rash from using DMSO.

Clean Skin

When using DMSO topically, make sure that the area of application is clean and there is nothing else on the skin, for whatever DMSO makes contact with potentially can be carried into the body. So, either wash the skin with a clean washcloth and soap and water, or take a shower before use. A good wash should always be your first step before using DMSO.

After exercising and if sweating, wash the sweat residue off the skin first before applying DMSO. The skin is porous and is an organ of elimination. Many wastes are removed through the skin, especially through sweat. You can assume that sweat contains toxins that should not be reabsorbed. To be on the safe side, shower after intense sweating before using DMSO.

I had a case of a woman who had a reaction to my DMSO hair regrowth spray (see Scalp Care and Hair Growth Formula in Chapter 6) after intense exercise. She had been using it with no concern for five days but then came back from a run and decided to use it while still sweating. She contacted me after her eyes became itchy and slightly swollen. After I ruled out other concerns, I deduced that she must have reabsorbed toxins through the skin from applying DMSO to her hair after sweating from exercise. It was a good lesson to understand both the power of the body to eliminate wastes and that of DMSO to carry them back in!

Mechanics who get grease on their hands, or anyone who works in an industry where residue can end up on the skin, must take great care to clean their hands properly. Washing with a pure coconut oil soap is very effective at cleaning grease, soot, or other grime from skin. If you prefer not to touch the DMSO directly or are applying it to someone else or to an animal and don't want to absorb any yourself, apply it with a natural bristle paint brush or organic cotton batten. Just make sure the paint brush bristles are natural and not synthetic, as DMSO dissolves many synthetic materials.

Detoxification Reactions

When starting DMSO use, it is wise to begin slowly. Once you get through the test patch successfully, you can begin to use DMSO according to the protocol best suited for your specific health condition (see Chapter 4). Your individual level of health or disease will determine your healing responses to DMSO.

I would also like to offer a note of caution to people who have been consuming chemicals in the form of processed foods, genetically modified organisms (GMOs), foods that were treated with pesticides/herbicides, alcohol, soda pop, caffeine, refined sugar, food dyes and other additives, or tobacco or cannabis. When they begin to use DMSO, or its derivative, methylsulfonylmethane (MSM, also called DMSO2), the rate that these chemicals are removed from the body increases. The liver is the primary organ responsible for eliminating toxins. Using high doses of DMSO when the body is filled with these toxins can overwhelm the liver's enzyme process. When this happens, secondary toxins can recirculate through the bloodstream and lymph system, fostering symptoms known as a healing crisis (see page 16). The symptoms include fatigue, bowel changes and bloating, nausea, headache, skin rashes, and mood changes. Sometimes, in highly toxic bodies, a healing crisis cannot be totally avoided, merely minimized. Drinking plenty of pure distilled or reverse osmosis water can reduce the effects to some degree. Ideally, resting and fasting will help the liver get the job done more efficiently.

So how do DMSO and MSM detoxify the body? The body uses the sulfur elements in these substances in a multitude of ways. One way is via the liver, which I've already mentioned above. The liver uses DMSO to create glutathione (GSH), a very powerful antioxidant comprising three amino acids, or tripeptide: glutamate, glycine, and cysteine. MSM, which is derived from DMSO, has been shown in one study to raise GSH levels by 80 percent, which benefits the body in many ways.[56] Deficiency of GSH puts cells and DNA at risk for oxidative damage.[57] When present at sufficient levels, GSH protects against free radical production, reduces chronic inflammation, supports heart health, and helps to remove heavy metals and other toxins from the body.

DMSO Odor

Pure DMSO has almost no odor, but when blended with other substances, the sulfur can be detected by our sense of smell. Once inside the body, DMSO begins to metabolize, or break down, which changes its constitution. When DMSO becomes DMS (dimethyl sulfide) through this breakdown process (called reduction), it gives off the sulfur-based odor that smells like garlic, onions, or oysters. Individuals metabolize DMSO differently depending on various factors, such as the water content in the body. Some people will not smell from DMSO while others can clear a room! I have heard many complaints about a spouse's breath or skin from using DMSO, though it is usually the breath that is the smelliest. Luckily, there are ways to work around this.

One suggestion I give is to use DMSO only on the skin and to use MSM internally (see Chapter 4 for details). Even though DMSO applied topically can be immediately tasted in the mouth, the DMS sulfur breakdown scent does not come through as much on the breath. Used orally, especially for gum or tooth infection, DMSO can cause a "rotten" smell. Still, using DMSO for a mouth infection can be a good idea despite the odor, because it stops bacterial growth. If the odor is offensive to you or others, I suggest doing the treatments at night before bed. By morning, the scent should have diminished.

Using wintergreen essential oil can also reduce or mask the scent of DMSO degrading in the body. I suggest creating a mouthwash by adding 1 drop of wintergreen oil to 1 ounce of water. Then, swish this mouthwash around in the mouth for about 30 seconds, and spit out. Do not swallow essential oils. You can use this mouthwash as needed to control odor. Make sure the oil you are using is 100 percent pure essential oil and not a fragrance oil or anything else synthetic.

I have another theory to offer. It's based on the two-stage oxidation chain that is carried out by enzyme systems in the body and results in MSM.[58] In the lab, one of the substances used to oxidize this reaction is hydrogen peroxide. My theory is that using a mouthwash made by adding 5 drops of 3 percent food-grade hydrogen peroxide to 1 ounce of pure water a few times a day while taking DMSO internally will encourage the oxidation process and reduce the odor. It may just save your marriage! Just be sure to never swallow food-grade hydrogen peroxide. Always spit it out.

What is fascinating about the odor of DMSO is not only variations in the individuals taking it but also variations of those around them smelling it. People with a higher level of copper in their blood have an increased awareness of the scent of sulfur. DMSO helps to balance excess copper in the body by encouraging the production of sulfur-containing amino acids and increasing glutathione levels. These bind and remove copper. Ideally, the more people around you taking DMSO, the better for everyone. If your family members are complaining about your odor but don't want to use DMSO, suggest that they start taking zinc, manganese, and iron, all of which complete with copper.

I am often asked about using odorless DMSO. All pure 99.995 percent DMSO is odorless; however, it is sometimes labeled as "odorless," so people think this means it won't make them smell when using it. This is not the case. Any company claiming their DMSO is "odorless" when used is misguided. As I explained above, as DMSO is metabolized in the body, its constitution is changed, resulting in the odor. No company can guarantee that this odor won't occur when your body metabolizes DMSO!

DMSO Taste

DMSO is an amazing molecule with so many benefits, but it is also a sulfur compound—and the flavor of sulfur is very bitter. I compare it to the taste of rubber bands. I know that does not sound so pleasant, but don't let it deter you. For all the benefits, it is certainly worth it.

I generally recommend diluting DMSO in distilled water and preservative-free aloe vera gel juice, although many of my customers and clients prefer to dilute the dose in either orange juice or grapefruit juice to mask the flavor. Some like to use tomato juice or grape juice. I have found that any citrus fruit or strong-tasting juice will work.

It is fascinating that DMSO can be tasted—and tasted almost immediately—when applied to the skin. Once the DMSO is in the bloodstream, it is in nearly every organ system within about an hour. The question remains, is the taste derived from blood absorption and circulation to the tongue and then to the nerves, or do the nerves transmit it directly to and from the brain?

Time-outs from DMSO

DMSO emanates from the skin pores for 24 to 48 hours and takes about seven days to fully clear from the body. Although the safety record of DMSO is impeccable, taking breaks is wise when using DMSO for the long term. These breaks allow for removal of metabolites and buildup from the body. If you are using DMSO every day, I suggest taking one day off each month. After six months of daily usage, take one week off to allow any residue to clear out. Another suggestion: At the start, use DMSO daily during weekdays and take weekends off.

Dose Precision

With DMSO, the dose does matter and successful use takes some self-education. I can imagine, as you read this book, that you already have gathered that notion. The percentages and applications of DMSO vary depending on the condition being treated. I have had clients tell me they were taking 3 drops of DMSO in a glass of water every day and not noticing any difference. Of course, they wouldn't see a difference; that dose is far too low. Drops are used in this manner only to enhance chlorine dioxide (CDS) absorption, as I will discuss later. I also have had people tell me they were using 99.995 percent DMSO on their skin and not seeing changes. This is because it is not the correct manner of application. For topical application, a dilution of 40 to 80 percent DMSO in pure water is needed for effect. For some disease states, the dose is lower while in others it is higher. This depends on the amount of water required for the DMSO to move into the tissues. For parts of the body with less water content, such as tendons, it is best to dilute DMSO further. I will help you sort out dosages in other chapters of this book.

In our modern, materialistic world, we tend to think that more is better. I ask you to put aside this thinking when it comes to certain medicines. Homeopathy is a classic example of "less is more," but this concept also applies to DMSO when it comes to percentages and dilutions. Remember, coming up with the correct dosage for your specific health concerns and being consistent will get you the best outcomes.

Use During Pregnancy

There is a limited amount of DMSO research in pregnancy, but as even small amounts of alcohol and caffeine can cause miscarriage or birth defects, it is prudent to avoid DMSO while pregnant. However,

I have known many who used MSM throughout their pregnancies, as I did in my own, with zero adverse effects. Even so, until we know more, it is a good idea to avoid both DMSO and MSM at this stage of our knowledge. It is okay to use DMSO if you are taking birth control and not trying to conceive. Because research on breastfeeding is similarly skimpy, it's best to avoid DMSO while breastfeeding. Due to the fact that DMSO is contained in some foods that we eat, small amounts of DMSO, for example in a skin cream with 20% DMSO or less, is acceptable for once-a-day use.

Risks for Children

I maintain that DMSO can be used on babies and children but in a limited capacity. Injecting children with DMSO or using the substance in high doses or for long stretches of time is not recommended. The evidence is not well established in this area.

In medical situations, DMSO is used to cryopreserve organs and stem cells for transplanting in children (as well as adults). However, high doses and injections of DMSO are not suitable for children as they have rapidly dividing nervous system tissue.[59] As well, transplanting DMSO cryopreserved stem cells into children can cause apoptosis (a type of cell death), or, in one case, reversible leukoencephalopathy (a disease that occurs in the white matter of the brain).[60] Note the part about the condition being reversible. Perhaps the DMSO was trying to protect the body from foreign cells that were doing other genetic damage to the body. The white matter edema was seen in a 16-year-old who had a large variety of chemotherapy agents in her bloodstream and had undergone surgery. Was her immune system properly functioning? Most likely not, as she was battling cancer. We can only speculate on these two cases, which are at odds with the incredible success we have seen with DMSO. For my own child, I have used DMSO in low doses, between 20 and 40 percent for topical use and 80 percent to control cavities, with great success and zero negative repercussions. I should note that my child was not taking any prescription drugs. However, when considering any change to your child's health regimen, be sure to consult a trained health practitioner first.

With Pharmaceutical Prescriptions

For the most part, a holistic approach to health and the use of pre-scription drugs are at odds with each other. A holistic approach works with the body, aiding it, listening to it, fueling it with nutrition, helping to direct what it already wants to do, detoxing, and supporting the organ systems. A conventional approach works against the body, working hard to stop its processes, mask symptoms, and cover up problems. Mixing pharmaceutical drugs with natural remedies can pose many risks either because they are working in opposite directions or their synergistic effect is too extreme.

For example, compare taking the pharmaceutical drug metformin for type 2 diabetes while detoxing the pancreas and liver (treatments in a holistic setting). Metformin damages these organs, but detoxing helps to repair them; these are conflicting, incompatible actions. Or compare taking antihypertensives to lower high blood pressure with taking vitamin C, omega-3 fatty acids, and magnesium to accom-plish the same goal. These nutrients naturally reduce blood viscosity, thereby lowering blood pressure in a gentle and natural way. However, mixing the antihypertensives with the nutrients may lower the blood pressure too much.

DMSO allows anything you are eating, drinking, or taking greater access inside the body. We don't yet know everything about this substance so we must always err on the side of caution, specifically when we are blending it with a pharmaceutical drug. On the other hand, blending DMSO with natural medicine seems to enhance the actions of vitamins, minerals, botanicals, and homeopathics, which are time tested as extremely safe. However, pharmaceutical drugs damage organ systems like the liver and kidneys as well as deplete nutrient resources, so this is where we tread lightly.

DMSO and Alcohol

First, I want to emphasize how important it is not to consume alcohol when using DMSO. Alcohol is a known carcinogen (class 1) and toxic to the liver, so drinking it is antithetical to the goal of improved health. Still, there is much to learn about DMSO in studying its interaction with alcohol.

A study conducted in the 1960s tested the effects of alcohol and DMSO in various combinations and found vastly different results based on the time in which each was taken.[61] This time, relationship is not only fascinating but also greatly informative. When alcohol and DMSO were taken at the same time, the DMSO protected the body from the damaging effects of the alcohol. In mice, lethal doses of alcohol were given simultaneously with DMSO, which reduced mortality from 50 to 37 percent. However, alcohol did not affect the lethal dose rate of DMSO when the tables were turned. So, the DMSO acted in a protective manner in the simultaneous time-relationship. However, when the body was given DMSO first, letting an hour pass before administering the lethal dose of alcohol, mortality was doubled. When alcohol was given first and DMSO an hour later, there was a four-fold increase in mortality. Timing is everything.

In another study, when DMSO and a small dose of cognac were taken at the same time, the garlic-like taste of the DMSO was completely gone.[62] This accidental finding led the researchers to understand that alcohol hampers the expiration of the metabolite DMS, inhibiting its formation when DMSO breaks down in the body. DMS is what causes breath odor. When alcohol was consumed one hour after DMSO was applied, it had the opposite effect—the odor and taste were even more pronounced. When alcohol is consumed and time passes before DMSO is taken, the odor of the alcohol dissipates from the respiratory air even though chemically it can still be found in the air. When DMSO is used first and then alcohol is taken, the DMSO inhibits liver alcohol dehydrogenase, an enzyme that breaks down the alcohol.[63]

DMSO has been used in veterinary medicine since the 1960s.[64] In fact, veterinarians were quite fascinated with the substance when it first arrived on the scene. There is a story from the late 1990s of a farm worker in my home province of Ontario, Canada, who used his bare hands to apply copious amounts of DMSO to horses over two days. Afterward, he consumed six to seven bottles of beer during a six-hour period. Normally, his body would have been able to break down the alcohol over those hours, but instead he was stopped by police for driving erratically and failed a Breathalyzer test. If this young man had been drinking more heavily, he could have experienced alcohol poisoning.[65] The moral of this story is, don't drink and use DMSO!

Note that DMSO affects other drugs, including insulin, corticosteroids, and atropine, in this same manner. When blended correctly, however, positive drug interactions can occur, requiring less drug and more access to the goal tissue or organ system.

Reactivity with Materials

DMSO will react with soft metals like aluminum but not with stainless steel. It will also react with copper, iron, or tin. Ensure that all jewelry worn does not touch the skin that has DMSO on it, unless the jewelry is gold or silver. Many jewelry clasps are made with alloys of nickel, so it is best to wipe off any excess DMSO on the skin and then wait 30 minutes before donning your bling. Of course, lead, mercury, cadmium, and other toxic metals should never be mixed with DMSO. DMSO can open the skin barrier to rust as well, so make sure you do your treatments well ahead of any gardening, building, painting, etc.

DMSO will dissolve certain plastics and is reactive with various substances such as certain types of silicone.[66] It is important not to mix DMSO with these materials. DMSO is safe or nonreactive with the following plastics:[67]

- High-density polyethylene (HDPE)
- Low-density polyethylene (LDPE)
- Nylon
- Polyethylene terephthalate ethylene (PETE)
- Polypropylene (PP)
- Polytetrafluoroethylene (PTFE)

DMSO is not compatible with or only partially compatible with:[68]

- Polycarbonate
- Polystyrene (PS)
- Polyvinyl chloride (PVC)—flexible and rigid

To generalize, most harder plastics do not react with DMSO, but softer plastics such as Styrofoam (a form of polystyrene) do react. Most manufacturers store pure 99.995 percent DMSO in glass. This is my preference. As a rule, I try to use glass for my recipes as much as makes sense. I do use PETE containers for DMSO combinations containing 25 percent or less DMSO, and when using polypropylene sprayers, a 50 percent solution is as high as I prefer to go.

If you have any silicone implants, I do not recommend using high doses of DMSO. Use it in low dosages and as far away from the implant site as possible. Although DMSO is only slightly reactive to silicone, it's best to be cautious.

For anyone who, in the past, has used Botox on the face or elsewhere, DMSO will heal the damage, disappearing the effect. If you currently use Botox, do not use DMSO!

Proper Storage

DMSO is light sensitive, so it is important to store it in a dark container if possible, or at least out of direct sunlight. A dark, cool cupboard away from other substances is a good idea.

The ideal storage temperature is between 59°F and 86°F. DMSO will freeze at 65.4°F so on a cold day in your house, you may find that your 99.995 percent pure DMSO has turned into beautiful crystals! Freezing will not alter or damage DMSO. However, if you want it at the ready, you will need to keep the temperature warm enough. I prefer to keep DMSO on the top of my refrigerator with a teapot cozy over it to protect it from light damage.

DMSO is hygroscopic, meaning it attracts water molecules to itself in a process called adsorption. This is another reason to store in an airtight glass container. If you leave DMSO in an open container, by the next morning the volume will have increased because the DMSO attracts water from the air.

Other Precautions

DMSO can speed wound healing and lessen scar tissue formation, although some people maintain it should not be used on infected wounds. In my extensive research I have been unable to find any evidence to warrant the avoidance. We know that DMSO is bacteriostatic, which means it stops bacterial growth, so there shouldn't be worry over the wound becoming infected by using DMSO. One Argentinian study found that DMSO used with antibiotic and anti-inflammatory agents was able to cure the majority of the test subjects' infected skin ulcers.[69] These results were very promising! Be sure to keep in mind that there can be some pain during application to deep wounds, but it soon resolves. When toxins from chemical burns, poison oak, or poison ivy are involved, there is potential for DMSO to allow access into the body. It is prudent not to use DMSO in these situations. There have also been warnings against its use on insect bites.

I have also had my own experience with using DMSO on infections. One man I worked with had an injury to the top of his foot. His shoe kept rubbing it, preventing it from healing, and it became so swollen and infected that he was unable to put his shoe on. I instructed him to apply a product that I make consisting of an 80 percent DMSO solution with added nutrients and aloe vera. He did so and informed me that the swelling reduced within an hour of application and by the next morning he could once again wear his shoe. The wound healed rapidly without a scar. He was very impressed with the level of healing he experienced, especially as the wound had been completely open.

When I first started to use DMSO, I applied an 80 percent DMSO formulation with aloe and added nutrients (containing iodine, vitamin C, MSM, the entire B vitamin complement, and magnesium) on my face and neck each night after washing. Within two days of use I had what I thought was a cyst or spot of acne open up on my neck, just over the parathyroid glands, which sit on the thyroid. I found it odd, as I'd never had such a blemish on my neck, but I just kept applying the DMSO. On the third day, this raised area got larger and then opened up and started to drain a curd-like material, which went on for around 10 days. I'd never experienced anything quite like it before. I wasn't alarmed but just stayed with it and kept applying the DMSO. It kept draining. There was never any pain and it never became infected. Then it stopped draining, began to heal, and after another few weeks completely resolved as if nothing had ever happened: no scar, no discoloration. I believe the DMSO allowed my parathyroid gland to express some kind of toxin and to heal itself directly through the skin, which, in this case, was the most efficient path of elimination. I marveled at this, one of my earliest experiences of DMSO, completely fascinated with a substance that somehow seemed to show a very high level of sophistication.

When I first started experimenting with DMSO, I learned another thing the hard way. I had rubbed a lot of it on my hands and then touched my tongue to taste it. In the next moment, I found myself in a position of cleaning rust off something, and somehow, I managed to get rust on my tongue within minutes of using the DMSO. I shook my head at my own silliness, but I learned something very valuable from this accidental experiment. I could taste the rust (from aluminum) in my mouth, and the tip of my tongue went numb. The DMSO had allowed the rust into my tissues! It is really that powerful of a substance. To counteract the numbing effects, I decided to consume a dilution of CDS in water, which ended up working for me. Fair warning that the FDA does not condone the use of CDS, but I encourage you to learn more about CDS by reading the research of Dr. Andreas Kalcker and Jim Humble and the experiences in the treatment of autism by Kerri Rivera. I know there are many readers of this book who have found DMSO because of CDS, and I truly believe that you have found two of the most effective remedies on the Earth with a broad range of applications! I encourage you to keep exploring and learning, and to keep sharing this important knowledge.

It is wise not to store DMSO in close proximity to any toxic substances as the DMSO could absorb that material. Also, do not store it next to iodine as it can "yellow" the DMSO. Avoid toxic substances, and make sure you are using all-natural cleaning products, makeup, lotions, etc.

There is no need to let fear keep you from using DMSO; just take precautions, make adjustments based on your own reactions, and allow time between the application of DMSO and the use of a questionable substance (like perfume or other non-natural beauty products). DMSO is absorbed within 10 minutes, but its effects on the skin barrier can remain anywhere from one to three hours, depending on your skin tone and type. This means that the barrier is more open to absorption. If you spill anything toxic on yourself by accident, immediately wash it off with water.

I also recommend avoiding the topical use of DMSO before swimming in a chlorinated pool. Pools are generally chlorinated with sodium hypochlorite or industrial bleach, which creates many metabolites during its breakdown. With the skin barrier open, the body is vulnerable to these toxic metabolites. After swimming in a pool, take a thorough shower and wait at least an hour before applying DMSO.

Reaction to DMSO

It is very important to immediately stop taking DMSO if you experience any symptoms of allergic reaction. This includes trouble breathing or shortness of breath, itching, facial swelling, rash, or hives. What these symptoms mean is that the body is unable to communicate properly and perform the functions that DMSO is encouraging. In this case, some detoxification is required before taking DMSO again. Imagine the body removing a toxin that has nowhere to go! What would happen? The body would have to identify the material as a poison and make sure it did not do further damage. It would need to bring blood to the area for this process to occur.

Histamine is a nitrogen-based compound that increases inflammation and is a vasodilator. It also acts as a neurotransmitter, communicating information to the nervous system. Your body is working to figure out the problem and to solve it quickly.

Some people create a lot of histamine, which can have a life-threatening effect. However, there is a simple, natural, antihistamine that you can make ahead of time if you are prone to allergies. This recipe comes from Dr. Janice Joneja, who has over 30 years' experience in the area of biochemical and immunological reactions related to food allergies and intolerances.[70]

Natural Antihistamine

2 tablespoons sodium bicarbonate (baking soda, not baking powder)

1 tablespoon potassium bicarbonate (available at most compounding pharmacies. Cream of tartar can be used if necessary)

Mix well and store in an airtight jar. To use, dissolve ½ teaspoon completely in warm water and drink it. Symptoms should resolve fairly rapidly. A second dose can be taken 20 to 30 minutes later if symptoms have not completely resolved. Do not repeat for 24 hours. This mixture can also be mixed into a paste, rubbed onto the skin, and left on the skin until it dissolves.

Note: Although baking soda is often used in detox baths, it is not commonly used with potassium bicarbonate. The inclusion of both in this recipe is important.

I hope you have enjoyed learning about DMSO in the previous chapters. You now should have a good grasp of DMSO, its properties, and its possibilities. I hope that you have begun to feel a sense of confidence about DMSO and how to safely apply it. Now, we will move on to protocols and recipes so you can begin to use DMSO in a confident and useful manner in many healing applications.

CHAPTER 4

How to Use DMSO

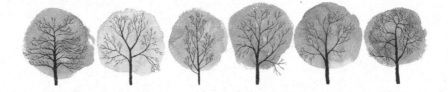

Well over 100,000 articles have been written on the medical uses of DMSO, and more than 30,000 citations can be found on PubMed.gov, a resource maintained by the U.S. National Library of Medicine, making DMSO one of the most studied substances we know. With all of this knowledge available, it's a shame that DMSO's benefits are still not widely known.

In this chapter, I focus on the use of DMSO for common ailments, but DMSO can be used across a wide variety of situations. In my case, I often think of DMSO immediately for almost any condition. DMSO is truly a powerful healer, but, for the best outcomes, it should be used with wisdom and knowledge.

There are many more protocols (a term that, in medicine, is often defined as a detailed plan for treatment) for DMSO's use than I have provided in this book. I've concentrated on the most common and the most important treatments, and included only some of the lesser known. Before you begin including DMSO in your at-home first aid treatments, it's important that you read everything thoroughly and make sure you understand the dosages and procedures. In addition, it's always best to consult your holistically trained doctor before making any changes to your health routine.

First, let's go over some preliminary pointers:

- You can make up many of the solutions I mention in this book in advance. Always label and date containers, preferably using a sticker and a permanent marker.

- Remember that DMSO can be used both externally and internally, especially if you are treating the inside of the mouth, stomach, esophagus, or the colon (in an enema, properly diluted), because it will be absorbed first through these tissues.

- To avoid oyster breath, I suggest taking ½ to 1 teaspoon of an MSM supplement (which you can find online or in most health food stores) every 12 hours orally and using DMSO topically.

- DMSO can be used topically in its pure state, but continued applications on the same area will thicken the skin and cause peeling. I generally do not recommend using such a high percentage. Please reference the "DMSO Concentrations Chart" on page 54 for more in-depth information on different percentages.

- Make sure the skin is clean and toxin free before applying DMSO. Either take a shower or clean the area with natural soap and water. If you feel you applied too much DMSO, wash the area with pure water (not tap water, unless it is filtered), which will remove any DMSO still on the skin. Do not wear clothing over a freshly treated area. Remember, DMSO is a powerful solvent, and it will take the dye right out of clothing and deposit it in the skin. Wait 20 minutes after applying DMSO to get dressed, and be sure to wipe off any leftover residue first.

- Do not wear synthetic fragrances (for example, perfume, cologne, body lotion, aftershave, hairspray, or fragrances left on clothing by laundry detergent or dryer sheets) when using DMSO. Synthetic fragrances are absorbed into the body through the skin, and you also breathe them in. Your goal is to benefit your health, so poisoning yourself with synthetic scents and materials as you are trying to heal is counterproductive.

- Do not consume any alcohol while using DMSO. If you smoke, limit your use of DMSO or quit smoking. Cigarettes contain over 4,000 chemicals, and negative interactions with DMSO are possible.

- You can use your hands, a natural bristle paint brush, a cotton swab or ball, or cotton batten to apply DMSO. Do not wear plastic or rubber gloves as DMSO will dissolve these materials. (If you want to wear gloves made of another material, test them first by soaking them in DMSO for 24 hours and checking for damage.) Also, do not wear nail polish when applying DMSO with your hands.

- Always start with a small amount of DMSO and patch-test your response. Work systematically up to the recommended dosage. You can use about 2 tablespoons or ½ ounce per day topically. Remember, more is not always better, but being consistent will get results.

- If you have any redness or a burning sensation, aloe vera is your friend. Have preservative-free aloe vera gel juice on hand to use in dilutions or to soothe the skin after topical applications of DMSO. Generally, a burning sensation occurs when the DMSO is blended with something else, like a nutrient or even salt from the skin.

- When you are using DMSO for pain, use it locally but make sure to apply it widely over the region, not only on the affected area. If you have an injury or a wound, apply DMSO right away as it can prevent ongoing damage from inflammation. This approach rapidly speeds healing, so for any ailment the sooner you use DMSO, the better.

DMSO Concentrations Chart

99.995%	Pharmaceutical-grade format should not be used in at-home first aid situations. Though it can be used purely on skin only for emergency situations, it should only be used with the help of a natural health practitioner. Redness, hives, and itchiness will be experienced. If used repeatedly on the same area of skin, the area will thicken, look leathery, and eventually peel. This is a side effect and once DMSO use is halted, the skin will return to normal, and often in a better condition than before.
90%	This is the strength often sold in health food stores either diluted with distilled water or with preservative-free aloe vera gel. At this strength, redness, burning, and itchiness can be experienced. It is also important to note that this percentage may be too strong for certain skin types. Repeated use at this strength can also lead to a thickened, leathery skin texture. Do not use this strength on delicate skin like on the face. As mentioned earlier, my usual recommended percentage range is 40 to 80 percent, and I would generally recommend avoiding applying a 90 percent strength concentration in at-home situations.
80%	This percentage is effective for skin applications blended with distilled water or preservative-free aloe vera gel juice. It is also an optimal percentage to use if mixing with other nutrients like vitamins, minerals, or botanical extracts. This is an ideal percentage for topical treatment of muscle injuries.

70%	Ideal for those who still find an 80 percent concentration too strong for topical use. Also excellent for making DMSO blends. Added to distilled water, this is a great percentage to use for pain and to help the DMSO penetrate deeper, as it uses water as a propeller to move deeper into tissues. This percentage or lower is best to use topically for tendons, ligaments, nerves, bone, or any region with less water content.
60%	Topical percentage for more delicate skin or those very sensitive to DMSO. Use similarly to the 70 and 80 percent dilutions.
50%	This is the maximum strength that should be used for the scalp, eyes and ears, ingested, and in a nebulizer. It can still feel very strong for these areas, so it is recommended to start with a weaker dilution first to test sensitivity or to slowly work up to a 50 percent dosage. This is also the maximum dose for oral use. Can be used on wounds and to assist hair to regrow or thicken.
40%	This dilution is safe for eyes (prepared in saline solution) and ears. I recommend this as a percentage for use on the face and other delicate skin.
30%	This dilution can also be used for the face, eyes, ears, and ingestion. Thirty percent DMSO in saline is a very good anti-inflammatory eye drop solution for the eyes.
20%	This is the beginner level for eye drops and ear drops. This percentage is also safe for animals and children and a great place to start to patch test for a sensitivity response.
10%	Use at this concentration if you wish to enhance the absorption of liquid formulas. At this low strength DMSO is not used therapeutically. At this concentration or less, it is used to mix with chlorine dioxide solution.

Aches and Pains

First and foremost, DMSO helps tremendously with pain. When people ask me about DMSO and its uses, one of the first things I tell them is that it is a powerful pain killer.

DMSO eases most types of pain: muscle pain, pain of injury, dental pain, nerve pain, pressure pain, and any pain caused by inflammation. This does not mean it will always work for every pain, each time. Results can vary and, of course, everyone's body is different. DMSO is best used in combination with another substance when it comes to treating pain; for example, partnering with CBD oil (cannabidiol, see page 83 for more information) for muscle pain and nausea or with the botanical wolfsbane *(Arnica montana)* to reduce muscle pain in a topical application. This is because, as we learned earlier while discussing the properties of DMSO, it is a transdermal agent that aids in the absorption of other substances.

For general muscle pain (such as soreness after a workout, or pain from being on your feet all day), I recommend arnica homeopathic 30CH or 30K and/or topical arnica salve as well as magnesium oil on the skin in addition to some gentle stretching. I also make a wonderful herbal combination with DMSO called Vein Tonic that assists with leg soreness and supports return blood flow.

For the pain of fibromyalgia (FM), I recommend starting with a very low dose. People with FM pain experience a detoxification response when starting DMSO that could make them feel worse at the beginning. Slow and steady wins the race in these situations. I usually recommend 1 teaspoon of a natural cream like my DMSO Peace Cream, which can be found on my website, containing about 10 to 15 percent DMSO for topical application two or three times a day. If it is well tolerated, more can be used.

People who have pain from shingles should be cautious and start slowly too, as DMSO can encourage a breakout because it helps the body remove toxins. In the case of shingles, sometimes the easiest route out is through the skin. As I tell all my clients, expression is healing. The body desires expression of what it does not want, and DMSO accommodates it. I personally believe that certain drugs or therapies merely act as a Band-Aid or suppress symptoms. Gently working with DMSO or MSM to help remove what the body wishes to expel is worth temporary discomfort; the chances of recurrence are slight or nil. In these cases, it is wise to work with a qualified medical practitioner who is familiar with DMSO and other natural therapies.

DMSO is a true analgesic (a pain-relieving substance), and its action is very quick. Some drugs that dull pain do so with side effects like drowsiness, loss of sensation, and nausea. DMSO causes none of these unwanted effects. Plus, the body does not create a buildup of tolerance for DMSO, so you do not need to keep increasing the dosage. In fact, I've found that it seems to do the opposite. Over time, less is required to get the job done. The length of time that DMSO relieves pain is approximately six hours. It is well suited for both chronic and acute pain, and the sooner the application, the better.

Make sure to apply DMSO, whether in a liquid, cream, or gel formulation, in a wider area than just the direct area of pain, as it works much better this way.

Burns

In my opinion, emergency rooms should be well stocked with DMSO for a variety of emergencies. Healing burns continues to be a huge challenge to modern medicine. When applied to the skin, DMSO has been shown to reduce pain, decrease swelling, and promote healing in both wounds and burns.[71] DMSO has local anesthetic effects, meaning it can block all sensations of pain. While you should imme-diately seek medical attention if you have been burned, DMSO aids in healing burns, as explained below.

DMSO can also mobilize skin tissue cells, improving injury to blocked or damaged blood vessels unable to carry oxygen.[72] Compromised blood supply is a problem because the longer that skin tissues are deprived of oxygen and nutrients, the greater the damage and the more time healing will take. In providing tissues with oxygen and reducing inflammatory response, DMSO speeds healing. Infections from burns, especially second- and third-degree burns, are also a concern. DMSO inhibits a wide range of bacteria and fungi that are attracted to damaged tissue.[73]

The DMSO Handbook for Doctors describes the case of a cook who was carrying a large pan of near-boiling grease that he spilled on himself. He had second-degree burns over much of his body. A solution of 50 percent DMSO with 50 percent preservative-free aloe vera gel juice was applied to the patient's burns immediately and then every hour for three hours. Afterward, it was applied in the same manner every eight hours for the next two days. The man recovered completely from the burns with no scarring.[74]

For minor sunburn, you can try using DMSO as first aid. A 50 percent solution diluted with water, colloidal silver, or preservative-free aloe vera can be used, as the skin is generally dehydrated and needs more water molecules for transport across the skin barrier. So too, the skin is sensitive, so having a more diluted solution is a good idea. Because DMSO can cause temporary burning and redness, keeping the percentage lower will minimize any stinging sensation. Many peo-ple find that topical DMSO applications are itchy for a time, and you want to minimize any itchiness when treating sunburn. It is always wise to apply DMSO to sun-damaged skin as soon as possible. The longer the delay, generally the longer the skin takes to heal. Using colloidal silver in sunburns is helpful to increase skin repair time and also helps to prevent scar tissue formation.

Headaches and Migraines

DMSO can prevent headaches and migraines. It is important to apply DMSO immediately at the first sign of head pain or the prodrome phase (early warning sign) of a migraine. Rub a 50 percent solution of DMSO in water, aloe gel juice, or aloe gel over the temples, between the eyes at the forehead, on the back of the neck, on the throat, and over the liver area. Apply about a 1 teaspoon amount every hour for a maximum of three hours. You might be wondering why I've recommended application over the liver area. This is because liver filters the totality of your blood volume every three to four minutes and is the master organ of the endocrine system, so treatment here supports the entire body. Your liver is under your right rib cage and spans across the abdomen, so try to apply the DMSO mixture on top of this area. You can stop applying the solution if the pain subsides before three hours. You can continue applying the mixture three times a day as needed. I also recommend drinking 1 teaspoon of DMSO diluted in 4 to 5 ounces of distilled water or juice right away; this will increase the levels of DMSO more rapidly in the body to help allay the headache and lessen the intensity of the migraine. As with all headaches, it's important to stay hydrated. Be sure to drink lots of pure, distilled, or reverse osmosis water. Fresh spring water is also acceptable. Be careful with drinking certain well waters as they can often contain inorganic minerals that can lead to arthritis and other health issues.

For full-body migraines or ocular migraines with pain, other measures must be taken. Magnesium is important. I suggest an internal dose in the 300 mg range and/or 10 to 15 sprays of a topical spray oil over unbroken skin every hour for the first three hours. DMSO also helps magnesium move through the skin faster thanks to its transdermal properties; however, topical magnesium is also transdermal of its own accord. You can also take a 20-minute full-body or foot bath with 1 cup of Epsom salts, 1 cup of baking soda, and 1 cup of Himalayan pink salt dissolved into the water to assist with the pain, placing a cold, damp cloth over the back of your neck and your forehead to prevent overheating the head area. Don't stay in the water too long as it can further exhaust the body.

Feverfew and passionflower are botanicals often used for migraine pain. Feverfew needs to be taken over a long period, one fresh leaf chewed daily over a period of months to see results. Some people also take it as a tincture. Passionflower is generally consumed as a tincture or a tea. These herbs have pain-relieving and anti-inflammatory effect, as does DMSO. Using a botanical medicine with DMSO creates a powerful and effective synergy.

Please do not use botanical medicine if you are taking any prescription drugs, as undesirable interactions could result. I generally help people come off the drugs first and then move to a natural protocol. Find a qualified natural medicine practitioner to help you transition.

Osteoarthritis

Many people with this condition use aspirin, an NSAID (a type of drug that reduces pain and inflammation), for pain relief. DMSO is also an NSAID, but it does not have the side effects that aspirin does. While aspirin can help reduce the pain of osteoarthritis, it cannot prevent the joint damage that occurs over time due to the condition.

For this specific condition, I suggest using both MSM and DMSO as well as magnesium and vitamins D and K2. For the pain, rub a 70 percent DMSO solution in distilled water or preservative-free aloe vera over the affected areas with a wide circumference two or three times a day. Take ½ teaspoon of pure MSM sulfur crystals twice a day (with or without food), or 2,000 mg of MSM in capsule form twice a day. The standard dosage of oral MSM is ½ to 3 teaspoons (2,000 to 12,000 mg) per day. When treating chronic illness, more may be necessary. MSM is also taken to support skin, hair, and nail health, and to assist muscle building.

For further osteoarthritis support, I recommend taking 5,000 IU of vitamin D (D3 or D2 for vegans) with 400 to 600 IU of vitamin K2 at dinner each day. Vitamin K2 helps deliver calcium into bones rather than tissues, and as of this text's publication, the Arthritis Foundation's website recommends the use of vitamin D to slow the progression of osteoarthritis and assist the immune system.

Another treatment I recommend is using 10 to 15 sprays of a topical magnesium oil over the affected areas twice a day right after applying DMSO, to facilitate magnesium's movement through the skin. An anti-inflammatory, magnesium is important for bone health, but its claim to fame is as a catalyst that speeds up enzyme reactions like metabolism or muscle building.

The larger joints, such as the hip, knee, and shoulder, may require longer treatment time. In really severe cases, DMSO injections (instead of applications to the skin) may be indicated.

Bursitis

DMSO has had excellent results in treating bursitis.[75] The body has 150 bursae, or fluid-filled sacs, that lubricate the areas where muscles and tendons slide over bone. The bursae in the shoulder, hip, elbow, and knee areas commonly inflame. Chronic bursitis can lead to calcium deposits that build up in the tendon. This most often occurs in bursitis of the shoulder and the hip.

Although DMSO can heal bursitis, it may require months of use. It is important to be consistent when using DMSO for chronic conditions. The general recommendation is to apply 5 mL of 80 percent solution to the damaged area and well beyond it two to four times daily, leave the solution on for 20 minutes, and then wipe off any residue.

Topical magnesium is also a good adjunct therapy as it helps to dissolve calcium. Vitamin C and castor oil heat packs over the area are also recommended; vitamin C is excellent for tissue repair, and castor oil is a deeply penetrating oil that helps to dissolve any crystallization in tissues. I have a few clients with bursitis who use DMSO on its own and have found it is not working fast enough for them, so I suggested these additions for a speedier result. They have been pleased with the progress of their healing.

Carpal Tunnel Syndrome

This syndrome is caused by the compression of the median nerve, which travels through the wrist. Many of the fingers and the thumb can become numb as a result. DMSO applied as a 50 percent solution in distilled water or preservative-free aloe vera gel juice two or three times daily can ease this type of pain, which is considered a complex regional pain syndrome.[76] In addition to the DMSO treatment, you can take vitamins. Dr. Jonathan Wright, M.D., a pioneer of natural medicine since the 1970s, suggests taking 100 milligrams of vitamin B6 (in P5P or pyridoxal-5-phosphate format) three times daily for several weeks.[77] If you'd rather go the topical route, you can crush a few B12 tablets, or open a capsule, blend it with the 50 percent DMSO solution, allow it to sit overnight and then apply it twice a day to the affected area. Just make sure the brand of vitamins you are using does not contain any dyes or flavoring. Applying the vitamin topically along with DMSO should help relieve the pain and also deliver the B12 to the local tissue via the bloodstream, encouraging more rapid repair.

Frozen Shoulder

In a person with frozen shoulder (the technical term is adhesive capsulitis), the shoulder capsule thickens and becomes stiff and tight, forming dense bands of tissue called adhesions. This condition—often linked to menopause, as 70 percent of patients are women over the age of 50—is characterized by stiffness, lack of mobility, and pain. A 70 percent solution of DMSO in distilled water can relieve pain and increase mobility when applied for up to a month. Because DMSO needs water to work properly, and there is less available in tendons and ligaments, healing can take longer than expected. Try to be patient! Apply the DMSO in a wide circumference over the area twice a day. In addition, I always recommend taking topical magnesium and vitamin C (buffered, 3,000 mg two to three times a day or higher) with any protocol dealing with skin, adhesions, arthritis, or inflammation. Each spray of magnesium contains 22 mg of magnesium chloride and you want ideally 10 sprays twice a day over the body.

I also advise to begin working with a topical, all-natural progesterone cream derived from wild yam. You can easily find these creams online. Using 100 mg progesterone twice a day will improve the cell-to-cell communication needed to accelerate healing of the shoulder. Employing DMSO, magnesium, vitamin C, and progesterone is a very successful treatment plan for frozen shoulder. I also would include 20-minute castor oil packs (see Chapter 5) over the affected shoulder daily to assist mobility and detoxification of the joint cavity. The magnesium can be applied after the DMSO to increase absorption rates.

Injuries

When it comes to treating injuries, DMSO has long proven to be an effective remedy. It's been used in sports medicine to treat strains, sprains, bruises, bone fractures, whiplash, and other athletic injuries, and also to treat injured horses. DMSO rapidly reduces inflammation and pain, increases circulation, and speeds the repair process. The results are even better when the treatment is applied soon after an injury.

Both the pain and swelling caused by an injury are usually resolved a few hours after DMSO application. Use a 70 to 80 percent solution or gel two to four times a day for rapid healing.

You may be skeptical about using DMSO to treat injuries, but it has always worked for me in the past. Once, I accidentally broke my index finger by catching it in my car door. I was in a rush and also tired, the perfect combination for injury. I was in so much pain that I was in a panic. Then I thought to use DMSO for my injury. After repeated application, within a week my finger had almost completely healed, save for a bump of what felt like marrow that had escaped from the bone. The DMSO slowly took down this little bump too. There have been absolutely no complications and my finger is perfectly repaired, almost as if the injury never happened. Please note that while this method worked for me, everybody's body is different. With major injuries it's always best to seek medical help before trying to heal the injury on your own. However, applying the DMSO as soon as possible is key to preventing a worsening situation, as it can halt the entire inflammation cycle that sets up at the beginning of an injury. This is why sports teams have it stocked at the sidelines to apply to the player as soon as the injury occurs. Oftentimes they are back on the field within a matter of minutes.

Tendinitis

The irritation or inflammation of a tendon occurs most commonly around the shoulders, elbows, wrists, knees, and ankles, as these are the joints we use most frequently. Applying DMSO regularly over a period of several months can aid in tendon repair and can certainly reduce the pain that comes along with tendinitis. However, there have been mixed results in studies of DMSO used for this condition. It is important to understand that the water content of tendons and cartilage is lower than it is in muscles. DMSO needs water to travel to the tissues, so the absorption of DMSO is lower in these regions. Moreover, there is limited blood flow to these areas, which also limits the reach of DMSO. This is why results can vary and the condition can take longer to heal than desired. It can be quite tricky to treat without a full holistic regimen. I suggest a similar healing approach to the frozen shoulder protocol, which uses multiple treatments within one plan.

Although studies found that 70 percent DMSO solutions don't seem to have a great outcome when it comes to tendinitis,[78] 80 percent solutions have been effective,[79] as have 90 percent solutions.[80] In the study looking at the 90 percent solution, DMSO was applied to the affected area every four hours. That rate was then decreased depending on how the individual responded to the solution. In some cases, the DMSO was applied for three weeks. All subjects in the 90 percent study reported fair, good, or excellent results, though there was some skin peeling seen due to using a high concentration. Keep in mind that a 90 percent concentration of DMSO is too strong for most skin types. It is best to use a 90 percent solution with the support of a holistic practitioner, in case you have any concerns and to make sure your healing is moving in a positive direction.

For even better results when using DMSO for tendinitis, work to increase blood flow to the area by first applying a hexane-free castor oil pack (see Chapter 5 for a more in-depth look at castor oil and DMSO) with a hot water bottle on top of the pack for 20 minutes. Wash off the area with a baking soda and water solution (dissolve 1 teaspoon of baking soda in ½ cup of water), and then when the skin is completely clean, apply an 80 percent concentration of DMSO. Leave the treated area open to the air for 15 to 20 minutes. When first beginning use, apply the DMSO to a wide circumference around the area of treatment every four to six hours and then two or three times a day afterward. In between applications, you can moisturize the skin with raw olive oil.

Head Trauma

The majority of head traumas occur in car accidents, sports accidents, slipping on ice, falling, and combat. In his book, Stanley Jacob stated the following about DMSO and closed head injuries: "DMSO … reduces swelling and improves blood supply to the brain. This improves blood oxygenation to brain tissue. Injured brain cells often aren't dead. When these cells get increased blood supply and more oxygen, and when the free radicals are scavenged, dying cells can recover, and brain swelling is reduced very rapidly."[81] Dr. Jacob noted that in studies conducted from 1978 to 1982, "We observed that when the human brain was treated with intravenously administered DMSO after a head injury, the swelling could be reduced within five minutes. No other treatment comes close to acting that quickly. In patients given other commonly used therapeutic agents such as intravenous barbiturates, the brain continued to swell. We've known about DMSO's efficacy for this type of injury for a long time."[82]

For most DMSO users, intravenous administration is not possible. In the situation of concussion or post-concussion syndrome, after consulting a medical professional, I advise the combination of DMSO topically and orally. Ingest 1 teaspoon of DMSO diluted in 5 ounces of juice or water twice a day for three or four days after injury, and then reduce use to once a day for three months. The therapy can be used for longer than this, using symptoms as a guide. Ideally, avoiding post-concussion syndrome is desired, so this is why the DMSO therapy should be used at length. Additionally, rub 1 to 2 teaspoons (5 to 10 mL) of 70 to 80 percent DMSO (diluted with distilled water or preservative-free aloe vera gel juice) two or three times a day over the temples, on the back and front of the neck, and to the tops and bottoms of both feet, making sure that all skin has been properly cleaned before application. It's also important to drink lots of distilled water. Taking magnesium and vitamin C supplements are also a good idea in this protocol, to aid the flow of blood and help the body remove free radicals.

Mental Health

Your mental health is extremely important and you should always consult your holistic therapist or properly trained psychologist before making changes to your mental health regimen. In this section we will focus on why DMSO might be helpful for certain mental conditions, but I will not provide any DMSO-based therapies as I've done for other conditions.

The first thing to note is that there is a strong link between inflammation and mental health issues. Danish researchers found a strong correlation between infection, autoimmune disorders, and mood disorders, supporting the hypothesis that depression is directly linked to inflammation.[83] Another study found that high levels of a by-product of inflammation, quinolinic acid, are associated with suicidal tendencies and chronic depression.[84]

Researchers at the Centre for Addiction and Mental Health's (CAMH) Campbell Family Mental Health Research Institute in Toronto,

Canada, scanned the brains of 20 patients with depression and 20 control participants with positron emission tomography (PET).[85] The scans showed statistically significant inflammation in the brains of those with depression, correlating the most depressed with the most inflammation. A 30 percent inflammatory increase was seen in those experiencing clinical depression. Another CAMH study showed that people with untreated depression for more than 10 years had higher brain inflammation than those who were treated.[86]

The reason why it's important to note the correlation between mental health issues and inflammation is because DMSO can act as an anti-inflammatory agent. One study found that DMSO was useful in treating various mental conditions like schizophrenia, manic depression, psychosis, delusional states, anxiety, and others.[87]

In this study, researchers observed 14 acute and 6 chronic patients with schizophrenia who were treated with intramuscular injections of 50 to 80 percent DMSO in saline. All patients were discharged from the hospital after 45 days. Three patients recovered completely within 15 days. One of them stated, "I have been out of my mind. I don't know what happened to me. I wonder what my children are going to say."[88] They all experienced a quick decrease in agitation, recession of persecution or paranoid feelings, a better tendency to communicate, a return to alertness, and a sense of calmness.

Eye Health

Ironically, it was the lens changes seen in the eyes of animals in DMSO studies that halted research in the 1960s. Later, it was shown that the same kind of damage did not occur in humans.[89] In the correct concentration, DMSO can be healing to eyes for most conditions. When it comes to eye problems, I prefer a 40 percent DMSO concentration as the upper limit. Research at the University of Oregon

Medical School in the early 1970s showed that 50 percent DMSO eye drops were effective in the treatment of retinitis pigmentosa (a genetic disorder that causes loss of vision) and macular degeneration. A 50 percent solution is used in an eye cup held onto the eye for 5 minutes, done once a day.

DMSO on its own or used with vitamin C and glutathione can assist with a variety of conditions including cataracts, glaucoma, eye injury, eyesight deficiencies like floaters or discolored sclera (the white part of the eye), retinitis pigmentosa, pink eye, and sties. Do not use DMSO inside the eye if you have a false lens from cataract replacement surgery, as the DMSO can blur the lens. Instead you can apply it over the skin of a closed eye twice a day.

Apply 1 drop of either 20, 30, or 40 percent DMSO solution in normal saline in each eye by leaning back and allowing the drop to roll into the eye from the inside corner. If you are in doubt of which concentration to use, always go low first. If you wear any kind of makeup, remove it completely with a nontoxic cleanser before using the DMSO eye solution. The solution will burn and sting, so have tissues handy. Over time, this response will lessen. The whites of the eyes (the sclera) may redden, but only temporarily. The aftereffect is generally refreshing and relieving. Apply drops up to three times a day as needed. For people who have had eye surgery like LASIK or cataract surgery, I recommend applying the DMSO solution around the eye socket instead of in the eye and also taking DMSO orally.

I had a successful case of a woman in her sixties with severe ocular pressure who years before had been diagnosed with glaucoma. She was on no medication and was a yoga instructor, so she was getting regular exercise. Under my direction, she used my 20 percent DMSO eye drops with vitamin C twice a day (she affectionately called them "liquid fire") among a variety of other homeopathic remedies. It took six months of treatment, but her ocular pressure returned to normal.

She was quite pleased and relieved, as the case seemed stubborn at first and she was feeling a little frustrated. I generally find that for every year of a disease, it takes three to four weeks of healing, so patience is essential.

Arthritis

Whether the joint pain is from osteoarthritis (OA), rheumatoid arthritis (RA), juvenile rheumatoid arthritis (JRA), or lupus arthritis, DMSO can be of service. It relieves pain and inflammation and improves joint mobility. It also manages amyloidosis, an excessive buildup of protein in organs seen in conjunction with RA.

One of the earliest studies on DMSO and arthritis, a clinical trial by the Japan Rheumatism Association in 1965, found that DMSO relieved joint pain and increased range of motion, although it did not have much success with swelling.[90] Various DMSO concentrations were used in this small study.

It is best to orally take 1 teaspoon of DMSO in 5 ounces of distilled water or juice once a day for arthritis. It is also a good idea to use the DMSO and vitamin C protocol (see page 89) for increased repair of the inflamed tissues. I also suggest the use of 10 to 15 sprays of topical magnesium twice a day. Another tip is to use warm castor oil packs over the afflicted joints before topical application of DMSO. When using DMSO topically for arthritis, anywhere from 50 to 80 percent DMSO can be used depending on the individual. If you are a DMSO beginner, I suggest starting on the low end of the concentration scale and working your way up once you see how your skin reacts to the substance.

Use up to 2 tablespoons (a half ounce) daily over troubled areas. Every 12 hours, you can also take 1 teaspoon of MSM sulfur crystals, which assist greatly with tissue integrity and detoxification. You could take powdered MSM in capsule format, but I prefer the larger crystals because they release more slowly into the system and also are more effective in killing parasites commonly found in the digestive tract. I find the best way to take the MSM is to gently pour the dose into the mouth and then drink it down with juice or water. Dissolving the crystals in water before drinking defeats the purpose of using them, and they are very bitter to take in this manner.

Restless Leg Syndrome

I have found that many cases of restless leg syndrome (RLS) seem to be improved by increasing the levels of magnesium, iron, or zinc. DMSO can increase circulation and assist the discomfort of restless legs, which generally worsens in the evening. It is interesting to note, from a Chinese medicine perspective, that health issues related to blood tend to heighten in the evening according to the principles of yin and yang. The evening is when yin rises, and all yin organs and matter become more active. Because blood is considered yin, any deficiency or issue with the blood will be more noticeable during the yin active time.

Before bed, apply 70 percent DMSO to clean legs and feet. Then apply magnesium oil liberally over the legs and let dry before getting into bed. It is best to take B vitamins in the morning as they provide energy but could keep you up at night if you take them too late in the day. Take 50 mg of zinc picolinate once a day with food as it can irritate the stomach. Ensure you are getting ample iron in your diet; take vitamin C to increase absorption of the iron.

Cavities

Your oral microbiome and your nutrition are the keys to preventing cavities. If the natural microflora (a.k.a. good bacteria) in your mouth has been damaged by antibacterial mouthwash, antibiotics, sugary sodas, tobacco, or alcohol, that can open the door to overgrowth of your own microbes (which act to remove damaged tissue) and foreign microbes (opportunists). When this overgrowth is coupled with eating poorly, it will create vitamin and mineral deficiencies and lead to further damage to the gut microbiome (intestinal bacteria), as well as an even larger issue: stagnation of the lymphatic system.

A lymphatic pump system moves through the major salivary gland (the parotid gland) and into the dentin (the hard tissue under the enamel that makes up the main part of a tooth). This pump system is responsible for the detoxification of the mouth as well as delivering nutrients to continue to regenerate, remineralize, and create fresh enamel. This pump system not only can stop working but also can actually allow microbes to be sucked inside and cause decay. As you can see, cavity prevention and repair is a whole-body affair.

To help strengthen bones and teeth, increase your intake of the fat-soluble vitamins A, E, D, and K2. Make sure to get plenty of magnesium and to drink lots of fresh, pure water. Eat fermented foods (for both K2 and good bacteria) or take a probiotic every day (I've found that the best method is to open a probiotic capsule right into the mouth). Brush your teeth with baking soda and activated charcoal or a clay-based toothpaste, and use 3 percent food-grade hydrogen peroxide as well as DMSO mouthwash (see page 100). Never swallow food-grade hydrogen peroxide unless properly diluted (beyond the scope of this book). Always spit it out and rinse your mouth thoroughly after use.

Muscle Repair

Turn to DMSO for help with muscle injury or even muscle wasting, which can occur in the elderly as well as people undergoing long-term health issues or stress. Apply 1 tablespoon of 50 to 70 percent DMSO solution over the injured muscles twice a day to help with blood flow and tissue repair. Take 4.5 to 5 g of the amino acid l-glutamine daily and ½ teaspoon of MSM sulfur twice a day. If you can afford it, it would be ideal to get a weekly professional massage or acupuncture to ensure the muscles stay in balance and to encourage optimal circulation. Hot and cold alternating hydrotherapy is also very valuable to speed healing to the muscles: apply a hot compress for three minutes followed by a cold compress for 30 seconds and rotate this five times, ending on cold, and then use a dry towel to friction rub the skin. This also has the added benefit of mobilizing the lymphatic system to remove cellular wastes more efficiently. Past the acute injury phase, it is important to start gentle exercise to the muscles to avoid imbalances, so taking advice from a good chiropractor or osteopathic doctor would also be wise.

Ears

DMSO can be of use for any ear issue, including infection, pain, blood clot, hearing loss, or tinnitus. It is also a good idea to treat the ears when dealing with a throat infection or sinus inflammation as the ear, nose, and throat are interconnected. A 20 percent solution is ideal for a child or an adult. The DMSO can be in a saline solution or pure distilled water. Apply 1 or 2 drops in the affected ear once a day. If you experience a sudden shooting ear pain from using DMSO, discontinue treatment for a day to let the ears respond appropriately. If there is any ongoing pain, discontinue the DMSO completely. Never put any liquid in the ear if there is an eardrum rupture. If you experience any fluid leaking from the ears visit your holistic practitioner and ask them to look inside with an otoscope to determine the status of the eardrum and if there is any cloudiness, tear, or bulging.

In traditional Chinese Medicine the ears are governed by the kidneys. If you have ongoing ear issues, it is advisable to support the kidneys to strengthen them. I usually recommend 1 cup of a strong infusion of parsley leaf and cornsilk tea daily and to detoxify the kidneys using a set of homeopathic drainage remedies (UNDA, Pascoe, and Pekana are companies that make such remedies) and using castor oil packs for 20 minutes three to four times a week. Make sure to apply a topical solution of DMSO over the low back area (where the kidneys sit).

Sinuses

Sinus rinses with diluted DMSO can assist with chronic or acute infections, allergies, dental issues, migraines, and eye pain. Make a saline solution in a neti pot (following the instructions with the neti pot). To begin, add about 20 drops of pure DMSO to the saline solution and see how it feels. If it burns at all, then reduce the concentration—but if it feels good, then you can either stick with 20 drops or try to use more DMSO. If your neti pot holds 100 mL, then 80 mL will be your saline solution and up to 20 mL will be your DMSO volume. Do not use more than 20mL of DMSO. Twenty-five to forty percent DMSO is your range to work with for sinus rinses. Remember to start with low doses of DMSO to test your tolerance. Also, the general rule in holistic medicine is to treat both sides, so even if you have a unilateral ear, nose, or sinus issue, treat bilaterally. This procedure greatly helps reduce swollen sinuses and helps to regenerate tissue that has been damaged by chronic inflammation.

Hair Growth

See my scalp care and hair growth formula on page 101. DMSO can help with hair growth by increasing circulation to the hair shaft. It also can eliminate hair mites that lead to hair loss. A 50 percent solution is high enough for hair and scalp use, but if you have sensitive skin, use 40 percent. Some people use it only once a week and others daily, but always use it on clean hair and after two washes if the hair is dyed. Please use only natural shampoos and conditioners. Make sure there is no product on the hair (gel, spray, mousse, etc.) when applying the solution. DMSO increases hair luster and thickness, encourages hair to grow longer, and stimulates new growth. The first thing that people notice when using a DMSO scalp treatment is that their hair stops falling out at the rate at which it did before the treatment. Remember, DMSO applied to the scalp travels into the tissues below because it is transdermal. Many people report that when using the hair growth formula they have better clarity of thought and their mood improves.

Skin Care

DMSO, in conjunction with an all-natural skin care regimen, is helpful for anti-aging, scar healing, reduction of wrinkles, and reduction of other blemishes, including acne. Be careful if you are using DMSO with any other skin care products, to avoid absorbing any toxins into the skin. I have developed safe, all-natural skin care products that either contain DMSO or can be used with DMSO to help anyone who is confused about which skin lotions, tonics, and creams are toxin free or which are not. Unfortunately, the skin care industry is not strict about toxins and many companies "green wash" their products, adding natural extracts into their formulations, making them appear to be natural when they are not.

For a general skin care treatment, it is best to use a 40 percent DMSO solution in distilled water or preservative-free aloe vera gel juice or less on the face, as higher doses can make the skin look wrinkled. The lines fade on their own, but that's not a desirable look, even if only temporary. Try a patch test before applying the solution to your entire face to make sure that your skin will react well to DMSO. Be sure that if you wear makeup, you have taken it completely off using a natural cleanser, and that your skin is completely clean before applying DMSO.

If you wish to treat your skin with DMSO before applying makeup, wait at least 20 minutes to do so. Most of the DMSO will have absorbed by then and the skin barriers will have closed up. If there is any remaining film on the skin after this time, simply wash your face with warm water and pat dry before applying your makeup. Some of the DMSO may have blended with your natural oils and did not fully absorb. I like to wash my face and apply my DMSO skin cream in the morning. By the time I am finished dressing and doing other morning activities, if I wish to use any makeup that day, my DMSO treatment is complete.

Hemorrhoids

Apply a combination of witch hazel and black tea or red raspberry leaf tea (all are astringents, which tighten slack skin) to a cotton pad and gently tap over hemorrhoids. Also, it is a good idea to drink red raspberry leaf tea daily because the root cause of hemorrhoids is the gastrointestinal system. Intermittent fasting is also a wise way to rest the organs of digestion during the healing time. Drinking 1 teaspoon of DMSO in 5 ounces of water or juice daily as well as applying a 40 percent DMSO solution over the hemorrhoids will help stimulate a rapid healing response. Apply the DMSO before the witch hazel and tea to increase delivery of the astringent. Continue the treatment for two weeks to ensure that deeper hemorrhoids heal fully.

Cold Sores and Persistent Shingles

DMSO often produces an interesting effect when used for cold sores just as it does for shingles (both are outbreaks of herpes in different locations on the body). It can encourage a full expression, meaning the shingles or cold sores will emerge, which is the process of the body removing the toxic material that has been residing in the nerve root. This is a healing response that should be encouraged; continue to apply DMSO until healing is complete. I've found that in some cases, consistent DMSO use can lead to a complete recovery from these outbreaks.

What I find interesting is that when I gather the history of the shingles patient, they usually have had an injury, a toxic exposure, or surgery over the area (called a dermatome) of the rash. Why do they have shingles exactly in that area? One woman only had the shingles express under her breasts where she used to wear an underwire bra. Another had it on her head where she experienced a closed head injury many years prior. Most of the time there are toxic metals and/ or scar tissue involved in these skin rashes. Detoxing the nerve is the main goal.

Post herpetic neuralgia is simply an unresolved shingles episode. When DMSO is used over these areas of the body this can lead to an increase in the rash temporarily as it detoxes/removes the unwanted material. Continue to apply the DMSO to help it successfully complete the healing process.

In a dropper bottle, combine a 30 percent solution of DMSO in 10 to 15 parts per million (ppm) colloidal silver (see page 86) or distilled water. I make a 50 percent colloidal silver and DMSO product that some customers have told me worked very well on their shingles or cold sores. Start always with the lower doses and go higher if you tolerate it well and want the healing to move along faster. Let it dissolve and apply over the affected region two or three times a day. I also advise taking 2,000 mg of vitamin C three times a day and a B-complex vitamin with food at breakfast every day to help with this treatment protocol.

First Aid and Wounds

Everyone should have *Arnica montana* in their first aid kits, both as a salve and in a homeopathic remedy. It can stop bruising and hemorrhaging, reduce pain, help with shock symptoms, and speed healing. For a wound or scrape, use Arnica first and wait to use DMSO until any bleeding is under control. DMSO can speed the healing of wounds, reduce pain and swelling, and support muscle, nerve, and other tissue repair. Having a low amount of DMSO (20 percent or so) in a salve or other healing formulation can allow for greater passage of the medicine in the salve or homeopathic remedy into the area of damage. For example, I make a fast-healing cream called DMSO Peace Cream that contains Arnica, St. John's wort, hemp, and DMSO. Make sure the wound is clean before applying any DMSO or other treatment. Using colloidal silver is a great way to clean the wound. Having a spray bottle of it handy in your first aid kit is a wise addition.

I have had a handful of cases in which children hurt themselves at play and the parents applied this cream to them soon after the injury. They reported that there was no bruising or swelling when there should have been and that the child had no pain or further issues.

Intravenous DMSO

In the states in which it is legal to do so, doctors have experimented with DMSO to treat the symptoms of cancer, atherosclerosis, Parkinson's disease, multiple sclerosis, and arthritis, with an intravenous push of up to 20 cc of a 25 percent solution of DMSO. An alternative method is to put 50 to 100 cc in 500 cc of saline or 5 percent dextrose, and drip it in over a two- to three-hour period with EDTA (a chelating agent that grabs certain molecules, like metals). Only doctors who are trained and experienced in this form of therapy should administer it. However it is always interesting to note the many possible avenues through which DMSO can be utilized as a healing treatment!

Conclusion

After reading through the many common ailments outlined above and how DMSO can be used to ease symptoms and heal injuries, I hope you are more informed about the many benefits of this incredible substance! You may have noticed that for some of the common ailments I have provided other natural treatments that work well along with the use of DMSO. There are many more ailments that DMSO can assist with that I have not mentioned here; if you are unsure, do some research and you should be able to find the correct doses and applications. Joining a DMSO education forum online is a great idea so that people who use it can share their experiences and learning can continue. The following chapter will go into greater detail about how DMSO blends with other substances and can give you some ideas on the marvelous synergy DMSO provides as a carrier and a solvent.

CHAPTER 5

DMSO Combinations

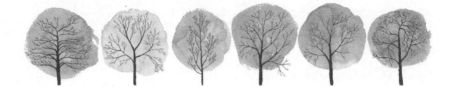

On its own, DMSO has unique properties and healing effects, but blended with other substances it reaches a whole new level. It works in synergy with other homeopathic and/or naturopathic treatments and medicines to maximize effectiveness. This chapter describes some healing combinations and remedies, many of them not well known. So too, as we learned earlier, it is unwise to take DMSO with prescription pharmaceuticals. It is best to come off these sorts of drugs completely before beginning any sort of DMSO treatment. I advise seeking the counsel of an educated professional if you're thinking about trying any of these approaches or making any changes to your prescriptions.

DMSO in Black Salve

Gentle drawing black salves are capable of removing splinters, embedded ticks, glass, insect bite venom, cactus spores, and other debris trapped just under the skin without causing dead tissue to form. DMSO is an essential ingredient in black salve. If you are interested in learning more about black salve, there is quite a bit of information available to you online, and I recommend you look into it.

DMSO with Essential Oils

DMSO is unique in that it can transport both water-soluble and oil-soluble molecules. Though there is a limit to the weight of molecules that DMSO can carry through skin layers, this still means we can use DMSO as a carrier for various applications. Even though essential oils tend to be larger or heavier than food nutrients (vitamins and minerals), in my experience DMSO will pull them into the body. I find there is more of a tingling sensation when essential oils pass through the skin. Please do not use these formulas on children or pregnant and nursing mothers.

Essential oils will slowly absorb through the skin naturally. They are generally applied blended with a carrier oil like sweet almond or grapeseed to avoid puddling of the essential oil on the skin, which can be irritating. Essential oils are volatile, meaning they easily evaporate. Blending with a carrier oil allows for proper dispersion and absorption without losing a lot of the essential oil to the air. DMSO can be used as an alternative carrier; blending an essential oil with DMSO increases the pace of absorption into the skin, reducing the amount lost to evaporation. Blending essential oils with DMSO also requires much less essential oil to get the job done. DMSO takes the essential oil much deeper into the tissue as well. This can help with deep infections or other pockets of toxicity (for example, in a joint space); the body will either clear it by dissolving it through the lymphatic system or else bring it to the surface to be expelled by the body. If your body responds in this way, note that the treatment is not causing an infection or an issue, but rather is removing a problem that was already present. It is best to continue to apply DMSO (without the essential oil) to prevent secondary infections and to facilitate drainage (for example, if a boil arises from the region). Many people mistake the effect for the cause, but the effect actually is the body healing.

COMMON ESSENTIAL OIL COMBINATIONS

Oil of Wintergreen: This is commonly used with DMSO to treat inflammation and pain. Please be cautious and use only 1 or 2 drops of essential oil in 10 drops of 80 percent DMSO per application. Those who have been diagnosed with liver disease should avoid wintergreen essential oil because the compound in it, methyl salicylate, must be processed through the liver. Also, anyone taking aspirin should avoid this oil, as both aspirin and the oil have blood-thinning properties.

Peppermint: Another popular combination is 1 drop of peppermint essential oil in 10 drops of 80 percent DMSO to rub over the temples to treat a headache or over a nerve inflammation like sciatica. If sitting in a car or at your desk for a long period of time is painful for you, this mixture can be a great help. It is also helpful for pain caused by osteoarthritis.

Black Pepper: Black pepper essential oil is helpful for the lymphatic system and is very warming. If you get swollen legs or your ankles retain water, try this excellent blend. Use 1 or 2 drops of the essential oil in 10 drops of 80 percent DMSO and rub that amount upward starting at the bottom of the leg. You will need to make this combination for each leg. There is great synergy between black pepper and DMSO, as both stimulate blood flow.

Sweet Birch: Sweet birch essential oil is a lovely muscle relaxant, as is clary sage. You can add 1 or 2 drops (or 1 drop of each) in 10 drops of 80 percent DMSO and massage the mixture into tight muscles up to twice a day.

DMSO with CBD

CBD oil is a cannabinoid derived from the cannabis plant. There is mounting scientific evidence that it helps to reduce pain and anxiety. With the opioid addiction crisis growing daily, we have a powerful combination at our hands blending CBD with DMSO. The male aspect of the cannabis plant is called hemp. The female plant carries the flowers and has THC, which gives the plant psychoactive properties when smoked or eaten. When THC and CBD are blended with DMSO and applied topically, the effect is different, but can still cause hallucinations in high doses. It also can increase sleep and dreams. I have been making a CBD blend with DMSO for many years that greatly assists pain and helps with relaxation. CBD is also of high value for treatment of the nervous system, such as with seizures, but has also been used successfully for MS, cancer, and many other diseases. Using DMSO with CBD will allow the CBD greater access to the cell receptors, causing healing cascades to occur.

Cannabinoids do still need to be detoxed by the liver (being fat soluble) so it is best to run a liver detox like a coffee enema or a homeopathic drainage remedy ahead of time. Castor oil packs over the liver for 20 minutes daily is a good idea, as well as using topical magnesium chloride twice a day to help the liver detox properly. The kidneys are also implicated, so staying well hydrated is also important. How many times have we seen someone experience dry mouth when they smoke pot? Be sure to drink lots of distilled, reverse osmosis, or fresh spring water!

There is an endocannabinoid system in the human body, which, simply put, is comprised of neurotransmitters, enzymes, and proteins and is an essential component of the central and peripheral nervous systems. Any plant that contains cannabinoids will affect these receptors. In addition to cannabis, we have black pepper, cacao, and echinacea, to name just a few. These cannabinoids get involved with multiple chemical intracellular pathways, regulate electrical channels, affect metabolism and energy as well as specific organelles called mito-chondria. This is a huge topic and we are still learning so much about this plant, its many varieties, dosages, and treatment approaches.

I have found over time that those who use cannabis recreationally are quite saturated with THC and CBD so when they use it topically or orally it is not as effective for their pain. The molecules can lin-ger on the receptors longer than the overt action is seen, especially if they are eating a diet of processed foods, smoking cigarettes, drinking alcohol, etc., their livers and kidneys are unable to clear the waste products made by the cannabinoids and the chemicals will be slowly excreted. I don't recommend abusing any plant and from my experience and training have learned that every plant has its healing dosage range. In my opinion using it topically or ingesting an extract is very effective, and smoking it comes with unwanted side effects. There is also evidence that children under the age of 25 can have irreversible brain damage from smoking cannabis habitually. The damage happens in adults too, but reverses when they stop smoking it, not so for those who were still developing their brains. Smoking cannabis via using specific doses and extracts, either topically or internally, has different effects and outcomes, which is important to know about.

How to Use DMSO with Cannabis Extract

Use a high-quality CBD extract in a liquid form blended with a 50 percent DMSO solution. Rub it over the temples at the side of the forehead, the back of the neck over the spine, and the bottom of freshly cleaned feet for maximum nervous system absorption. Start with 15 ml of total liquid volume and see how you feel. If you are groggy the next day, you may need to do a liver detox as I have already mentioned, or you might need to apply it earlier in the evening and use less of the mixture.

If you wish to blend THC and CBD cannabis with DMSO, find a heavy CBD leaning strain (a cannabis designed to have less THC and more CBD). I make an oil extraction of the dried plant as I would extract any plant for any of my medicinal topical products and then also make a DMSO extract also of dried plant material. The DMSO will absorb the water-soluble aspects of the plant and the oil will absorb the fat-soluble components. Mixed together this is a powerful and potent blend to reduce anxiety and produce a sense of calmness. The effects are generally immediate so please use caution on your dosages if you blend DMSO with cannabis in any form.

DMSO with Castor Oil

Castor oil has amazing properties and is one of the most highly penetrating oils on Earth. Consider the synergy between such a penetrating oil and transdermal DMSO, which is highly penetrating itself. The possibilities are incredible!

Properly prepared castor oil is hexane free and contains undecylenic acid, which is a very effective antifungal agent.[91] Castor oil used on its own provides so many benefits: It softens masses, detoxifies organ systems, and helps to remove crystallized calcium deposits in arthritic joints. For detox, I generally advise daily 20-minute applications of castor oil packs (you can make your own by soaking a piece of wool flannel or cotton cloth in castor oil) with heat (like a hot water bottle placed on top of the pack). It is always important when encouraging detoxification to drink plenty of pure water, 8 to 12 cups (2 to 3 liters daily), to flush out toxins and to stay hydrated. And remember, it has to be water—juice, tea, and other beverages don't act the same way as water.

The combination of DMSO and castor oil is excellent for all rheumatic complaints, pain, stiffness, injury, scar tissue formation, and other growths. I have had clients report rapid healing of tendons, strengthening of joints, and reduction of pain, including bone spur pain. Please do not use this treatment on cancerous tumors. Women should not use castor oil when menstruating, pregnant, or nursing.

How to Use DMSO with Castor Oil

Apply a thin layer of castor oil over the treatment area, making sure the skin is clean and dry. Then pat on an 80 to 90 percent DMSO over the oil and let it work in for about 10 minutes. Earlier in this book I did mention that an 80 percent concentration of DMSO should be the maximum percentage for at-home use. However, when used in this situation, the castor oil will dilute the DMSO to a level that will not burn or dry out the skin. If you are concerned about how your skin might react to a higher percentage of DMSO, feel free to use a lower concentration. Keep in mind that castor oil stains fabrics, so after treating the feet you can put on clean cotton socks (either organic cotton or well-washed if conventional cotton), if you want to move around freely. Either leave the mixture on the skin or, after about 20 to 30 minutes, wash off the oily residue with baking soda solution (dissolve 1 teaspoon of baking soda in ½ cup of water). You do not need to add heat as the DMSO will warm up the castor oil on its own, but you can place a hot water bottle wrapped in a tea towel on your feet if you like.

DMSO with Colloidal Silver

Homeopathic and naturopathic practitioners believe that colloidal silver is a powerful and natural antibiotic that does not give rise to resistance as antibiotics do. It comes in a variety of strengths and most people take it orally as a supplement or apply it topically on their skin.

Colloidal silver used with DMSO is a potent combination, given DMSO's nature. Along with amplifying substances and giving them greater access to tissues, DMSO is bacteriostatic (meaning it inhibits bacteria). This combination can be used to deal with any level of infection systemically or topically.

How to Use DMSO with Colloidal Silver

Mix pure, pharmaceutical-grade DMSO with 10 to 15 ppm of colloidal silver in a 50:50 ratio for use as a mouthwash, for topical wounds (infected or not). Be sure to spit out the mixture thoroughly after you are done using the mouthwash. You can also add this 50:50 mixture to a saline solution to flush sinuses. Place 5 mL of this 50:50 mixture into 2 ounces of distilled water to drink for any stomach or intestinal concerns; for example, stomach infections, small intestine bacterial overgrowth (SIBO), or ulcers.

DMSO with Botanical Medicine

Botanical medicine needs to be prepared so that we can extract the components of the plant (called constituents) for therapeutic effects. One of the most common solvents used with botanical medicine is simply water. We make teas (called infusions), we simmer them on a heat source for longer periods of time (called a decoction), we let them sit and ferment or we soak them in a cloth to apply to the body (called a liniment).

Using water will extract the water-based components of the plant. We also use alcohol as a solvent with herbs, and when we do this, we make something called a tincture. Alcohol will remove both water-based and oil-based components in a protic manner, which means it uses hydrogen bonds and lends a proton in its chemical reaction to grab hold of the herbal material.

Oil-based extractions of herbs are used mainly for topical applications. I make many skin-healing salves, oils, and creams using this extraction method, as well as garlic, mullein flower ear oil that gets fantastic feedback. The oil is added to the dry or slightly wilted fresh herbal material and gently warmed, either on the stove, inside the stove, or in the sun. The nice aspect about sun-transferred botanical medicine is that the UV will reduce the bacterial population; however, it is a slower process, taking many weeks to finish extracting. Even so, it is the method I most prefer and use in the summer months.

DMSO is also an excellent solvent as you have learned. Using DMSO as a soaking medium for botanical medicine is not well known or commonly used. However, DMSO is aprotic (the opposite of alcohol) so when forming the chemical reactions it will form a different bond structure than alcohol (for you chemistry geeks: DMSO gives a 1,4 addition while alcohol gives a 1,2 addition). So far, I have extracted a multitude of herbs using DMSO as the prime solvent, including cannabis, St. Johns wort, *Arnica montana*, calendula, horsetail, cayenne pepper, dandelion root and leaf, burdock root, and many more. I have used all of these on my skin with great success. I find the transdermal action of the herbs and the subsequent results are greater with DMSO than using an oil extract. I prefer to combine oil extracts and DMSO extracts together for added synergy. This is an area that deserves plenty of focus and study but is largely unexplored.

There is actually a relationship between solvents and transdermal action. Many of the transdermal chemicals I have listed in Chapter 8 are also solvents. A solvent will dissolve the material it is paired with and break down the cellular material so that the components are floating inside the solvent liquid. Many laboratories and industries use solvents in varying fashion to isolate a component of something they are studying or using to create a product. This topic can get quite chemistry laden, but the takeaway is that you can use DMSO to extract botanical medicine. However, unless you understand both the plants and are knowledgeable enough to use chemistry principles to predict the outcome, it is best left for the experts.

DMSO with Vitamin C

DMSO with vitamin C can be used as a specific cancer protocol. If you have recently been diagnosed with cancer, I suggest that you do an internet search for the details of this protocol and educate yourself on the pros and cons. Please do NOT do this if you have advanced cancer. Here I am going to talk about cancer prevention using this blend.

Our body makes cancer cells every day. When we have a healthy, functioning lymphatic system and microbial terrain, our body can repair or replace damaged cells with ease. The cells of our body use glucose as a fuel, which is readily taken into the cell by insulin. Vitamin C closely mimics glucose and is equally invited into the cells. Combining DMSO with vitamin C allows for greater absorption of the vitamin C into cells.

Ascorbic acid is an inactive form of vitamin C that is unbound to a mineral and can be used in small doses with DMSO, for example if you feel you are starting to come down with a cold. It will just use your existing minerals to activate; as well, your own antioxidants will be used during liver metabolism. However, when taking larger doses of vitamin C, it is important to use a buffered form and a product that also contains an antioxidant like acai berries, wild blueberries, strawberries, etc. Fruits are primarily antioxidants.

Potassium ascorbate, calcium ascorbate, or sodium ascorbate are the most common buffered, mineral bound, activated vitamin C formats you will find for sale. I personally prefer sodium ascorbate; however, those who have cancer should limit their sodium intake, even though the sodium cleaved from the ascorbate is not used by the body in the same way as is sodium chloride, or regular salt. For example, it will not increase blood pressure, so it is safe to use in hypertensive people.

Regardless, I suggest using a calcium ascorbate with about 15 percent potassium ascorbate, even if the product has some ascorbic acid involved, for those with early-stage cancer. I recommend adding the powder to water and consuming it orally to trigger the limbic system and prepare the body for optimal absorption.

How to Use DMSO with Vitamin C

Note: For this combination to work properly, it is important to be eating a whole foods diet, removing any other sugar intake, synthetic sugars, white rice, potatoes, white bread, soda, etc. You want the cells to be encouraged to use the vitamin C as it would sugar.

Take 5 grams of vitamin C in the buffered format twice a day. You can find vitamin C in powder form easily online or in health food stores. Drink 1 teaspoon of pure 99.995 percent DMSO (be sure to work up to this dosage slowly, method explained below) diluted in 5 ounces of distilled water or juice 10 minutes before the second dose of vitamin C. You must take this DMSO dose on an empty stomach, two hours after your last meal and not eat for two hours after you take the dose. The DMSO will also help the vitamin C absorb better into the body, specifically across the cellular membrane.

DMSO should always be worked up to the desired dosage slowly, especially on an empty stomach. Start with ¼ teaspoon in 5 ounces of distilled water or juice the first day, ½ teaspoon in 5 ounces the second day, ¼ teaspoon in 5 ounces the third day, and 1 teaspoon in 5 ounces the fourth day and onward. If you have any discomfort in the abdomen, do not increase the dose and let it work on the gastrointestinal system gently for a little while. Then when those symptoms clear up, you can increase the dose. To stop this protocol, it is best to taper off, reducing the amounts by half and half again.

Use this protocol for two weeks, four times a year, ideally around the time the seasons change. This will also help to gently detox the body and prevent colds and flus by encouraging proper elimination of wastes.

DMSO with MSM

MSM (methylsulfonylmethane) is a chemical that can be found in a variety of plants, as well as animals. Interestingly, one of the plants I have mentioned a few times now, horsetail (*Equisetum arvense*) contains high levels of MSM. It comes in powder form and you can find it easily online, sometimes called organic sulfur. It is made from DMSO in a laboratory. Most people take MSM to try to relieve the swelling and pain caused by tendinitis, rheumatoid arthritis, or osteoarthritis. It primarily assists with collagen synthesis, forming skin, blood vessels, and hair and strengthening nails. What's great about MSM is that there are no known side effects that come along with taking it. It is also a bonus that, unlike DMSO, there is no oyster or garlic smell on the skin or breath afterward.

When a person uses DMSO, 15 percent of it is converted into MSM, also called DMSO2, as it oxidizes. You might be wondering why the two should be used together, as DMSO basically turns into MSM in the body. One reason is to obtain all the sulfur-enriching benefits without the DMSO smell. MSM and DMSO together are excellent for supporting more serious conditions like Lyme disease, lupus, and cancer. The Independent Cancer Research Foundation is researching the use of DMSO with substances other than chemotherapy. One study showed MSM in vitro reversed a melanoma cancer cell into a normal cell.[92] Partnered with DMSO, MSM can have greater access to cancer cells. Though research is still in the early stages, I am excited to see what further advancements are made. There are already certain protocols combining DMSO and MSM with vitamin C and chlorine dioxide solution, as well as other substances, called DMSO Potentiation Therapy.

How to Use DMSO with MSM

Always start with a low dose and work up to avoid or reduce any uncomfortable detoxification symptoms. Start with 500 mg of MSM in either a powder or capsule format twice a day. There are around 4 grams (4,000 mg) in a teaspoon. Most MSM capsules are between 500 to 1,500 mg per capsule. Work up slowly over a few days to ½ teaspoon twice a day. For treating something specific, take 1 teaspoon twice a day. This can be taken with or without food. I have found no ill effects from taking it on an empty stomach.

You can also take both MSM and DMSO internally together to increase the absorption of the MSM and to decrease the amount of MSM that the DMSO makes so you can take less DMSO for the same effect. Take ½ to 1 teaspoon of DMSO diluted in 5 ounces of water or juice followed by the dose of MSM that you have worked up to, for example 1 teaspoon. I like to use the MSM in crystal format. They look like large bath salts. I place the dry MSM on my tongue and drink it down with some organic juice.

This is also a great protocol when working to kill parasites as the DMSO will help to open up access for the MSM to reach and make life very uncomfortable for those little critters, at the same time assisting repair of the gut lining. You should start to see hair, nails, skin, and digestion improving from using MSM and DMSO in this way, within a week or two.

CHAPTER 6

DMSO Recipes

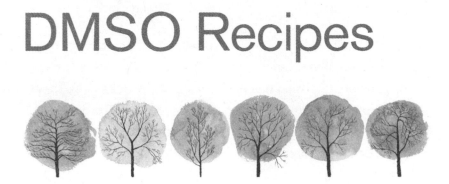

In preparation to write this book, I bought just about every DMSO book I could find. Not one of them had specific DMSO recipe blends that you could make at home. This chapter, as well as the previous one, discusses DMSO in combination with other natural remedies. To my knowledge, this is new information about DMSO and not available in any other book or with a simple internet search. Some of the combinations I offer are adaptations, others completely new. I designed combinations using my knowledge of plants, my chemistry background, my experience formulating medicines, and the personal and professional use of these blends I acquired over many years. Please respect the wisdom these precious recipes contain. It is my wish that you feel confident enough to use them for any health situation and that this section becomes filled with notes, bookmarks, and dog-ears, a valued book that will be handed down from generation to generation. As with any and all changes you plan to make to your health regimen, be sure to talk with your holistically trained doctor before incorporating anything new.

Antifungal Drops

100 mL glass dropper bottle

1 mL Lugol's iodine or povidone-iodine

44 mL 99.995 percent pharmaceutical-grade DMSO

55 mL distilled water

These drops will work wonders on toenail fungus and other fungal issues such as athlete's foot, jock itch, and candida blooms (for example, on areas of skin that touch, like under the breasts). They also work on fungal issues in animals, especially in dogs during humid weather or that are chronically wet from constant swimming or whose ears don't dry properly.

To the clean dropper bottle, add the iodine, DMSO, and distilled water. Screw on the top and shake until mixed. Store at room temperature in a dark cupboard.

For nail fungus: Wash the skin and nails well with a nontoxic soap. Apply 1 to 2 antifungal drops (just enough to cover the nail on top and underneath) twice daily to the nail, under the nail plate, and on the surrounding skin. Up to six months may be needed for complete healing.

For athlete's foot: Soak the feet in a 50 percent solution of apple cider vinegar and water for five minutes, then dry well. Apply 1 to 2 antifungal drops (just enough to cover the nail on top and underneath) between the toes and on all affected areas of skin twice a day until resolved. If possible, clean athletic shoes in the washing machine, or replace old shoes to avoid reinfection.

Analgesic Formula

50 mL glass dropper bottle	30 dried cloves
Mortar and pestle or zip-top bag and rolling pin	99.995 percent pharmaceutical-grade DMSO

Both DMSO and cloves have analgesic properties, and soaking cloves in DMSO greatly enhances these properties. This analgesic formula is excellent for toothaches, muscle pain, and nerve pain.

Slightly break 30 cloves with a mortar and pestle or zip-top bag and rolling pin. Add the broken cloves to the glass bottle. Add DMSO to cover the cloves, leaving some space for agitation and the glass dropper. Shake daily for seven days. Then strain out the cloves and return the liquid to the bottle. You can top up the DMSO if you wish. Store at room temperature in a dark location.

For tooth pain: Apply 1 or 2 drops on the affected area two to three times a day or as needed for pain. You may need to apply a few drops every 15 minutes until you reach the desired effect. If you don't find relief after an hour, you will need to take other measures.

For muscle or nerve pain: Place 14 drops of the formula in a small glass bowl or glass measuring cup, and add 6 drops of pure distilled water or preservative-free aloe vera gel juice. Apply the entire mixture to clean skin in the affected area up to four times daily.

For use with black salve: To a glass container, add 1 tablespoon of the formula, 3 drops of pure eucalyptus essential oil, 3 drops of pure camphor essential oil, 2 drops of Lugol's iodine or povidone-iodine, and 1 teaspoon of pure gum turpentine. Mix well and apply the mixture to the skin before applying black salve. Applying this entire solution to the skin before using black salve will increase the likelihood that the salve "takes" much better, as sometimes the salve does not absorb very well on first application.

Eye Drops

30 mL glass dropper bottle

118 mL distilled water

¼ teaspoon pure, natural sea salt (noniodized)

6.25 mL 99.995 percent pharmaceutical-grade DMSO

The eye has a microbiome, or community of microorganisms, that acts as a natural immune system.[93] When making these eye drops, use the sterile technique described below, to avoid bacterial contamination of the drops. We want to preserve the good bacteria in our eyes and avoid upsetting the microbiome balance by introducing new or foreign bacteria.

Disassemble all parts of the dropper bottle. Bring a pot of water to a boil and lower the bottle pieces gently into the water with tongs or a spoon. Let the pieces boil for five minutes, then remove them and place them on a clean towel or drying rack to air-dry. Reassemble the dry pieces with clean hands or wear clean gloves. Keep the lid capped while you make the solution to avoid air contamination.

In a pot, place the distilled water and natural sea salt, and heat gently until the salt has dissolved. Using a syringe, add the DMSO to the dropper bottle. Then add 23.75 mL of the saline solution you just made to the bottle, replace the cap, and shake. There will be leftover saline solution in the pot, which you can discard. The mixture will become hot in the glass dropper bottle due to the exothermic (heat-producing) reaction of DMSO with water. You have just made a 20 percent DMSO saline eye solution. (To make a 40 percent solution, simply double the dose of DMSO and subtract the amount from the saline content.) Label and date your bottle; you should make a new solution after six months.

To be as clean as possible when using the eye drops, please wash your hands with soap and hot water, and dry them with a clean towel before using the eye dropper. Make sure not to touch the eye area with the tip of the dropper as this will contaminate it. If you accidentally do this, be sure to wash the dropper in hot, soapy water and dry it with a clean paper towel or freshly washed towel.

I make these drops and they are available in my store (see page 102) if you prefer to purchase them ready-made. Also note that, in a pinch, the 20 percent solution can work as ear drops; however, I recommend following my ear drops formula below.

Ear Drops

50 mL glass dropper bottle

45 mL 15 ppm colloidal silver

5 mL 99.995 percent pharmaceutical-grade DMSO

This ear drop formula makes a solution containing 10 percent DMSO with 90 percent colloidal silver solution. Add the DMSO and colloidal silver to the clean glass dropper bottle. Cap and gently shake. Wait for the exothermic (heat-producing) reaction to complete before using. Apply 1 or 2 drops in each ear one to two times daily for a week. When symptoms disappear, continue treatment a few days longer to ensure that the problem doesn't return. Make sure to label and date your bottle. You should make a new solution after six months.

Sinus Rinse

Neti pot or metered
nasal tip applicator

8 ounces distilled water

¼ teaspoon neti salt or
noniodized sea salt

11 mL 99.995 percent
pharmaceutical-grade DMSO

½ teaspoon 15 ppm
colloidal silver

½ teaspoon preservative-free
aloe vera gel juice (optional)

For a sinus rinse to manage sinus infections, polyps, injuries, allergies, or general inflammation, a 5 to 10 percent DMSO solution is ideal. Do not use this solution if the inside of your nose is raw or bleeding.

You can purchase a neti pot or use a glass to "sniff" in the water. Alternatively, you can purchase a product that has a metered nasal tip applicator and make a solution in that bottle. Any of these items can be found easily online.

Use lukewarm distilled water when making this rinse to prevent bacterial contamination. If you only have access to tap water, boil the water for three minutes first and allow it to cool until it is lukewarm. Add the neti salt or noniodized sea salt to the lukewarm water. Stir until fully dissolved. Add the DMSO to the solution. Then add the colloidal silver using a plastic or wooden spoon (not metal). Stir gently. The mixture is now ready for you to rinse both sinuses. If the rinse stings too much, add ½ teaspoon of preservative-free aloe vera gel juice to help to soothe the sinus tissues.

Wound Spray

100 mL glass spray bottle

50 mL 99.995 percent
pharmaceutical-grade DMSO

50 mL distilled water or
15 ppm colloidal silver

I want to tell you the story of the time my daughter learned to ride her bicycle without training wheels. She is a very bold and confident child (very much like her mother) and sometimes can be overconfident. Before we had a chance to purchase knee and elbow pads, she wanted to ride down the lane with her friends. She slipped on a patch of sand and over she went, scraping her knee quite badly. It is a lesson I think we have all had at some point in our childhood.

At first, I didn't think to use DMSO on the wound. I just cleaned it, sprayed it with colloidal silver, and applied a homemade calendula salve. However, the wound was taking a lot longer to heal than we wanted, and it was still causing her pain. I asked her if she would be okay if I sprayed a 50 percent DMSO solution on her open wound, even if it might sting. She agreed and we tried it. It turned out that the DMSO did not sting at all! She found immediate relief from the spray and so we decided to apply it three times a day. The next day a proper scab had formed but she complained that it felt tight, so I moistened it with the calendula salve over the next two to three days. It healed very quickly, the new skin came in beautifully, and there was no scar.

I make this wound spray for my customers and it is well loved. Using a funnel, pour the DMSO and distilled water into the spray bottle. You can also choose to use 50 mL of 15 ppm colloidal silver in place of the water if you prefer. Store the spray in a cool, dry place and make a new batch after six months. You can use this formula on all kinds of wounds, but it is best to wait to use DMSO until the wound has stopped bleeding. Avoid using this on surgical wounds, as the sutures could be dissolved by the spray.

Mouthwash

3.5 mL 99.995 percent pharmaceutical-grade DMSO

3.5 mL 3 percent food-grade hydrogen peroxide

7 mL distilled water or distilled water mixed 50-50 with preservative-free aloe vera gel juice

Here's a mouthwash that you can use to treat symptoms of gum disease and tooth infections, although always see your dentist as soon as possible for serious dental issues. I personally advise my clients to find a biological, mercury-free, and mercury-safe dentist in their area. Combine the DMSO, hydrogen peroxide, and distilled water (or distilled water mixed with aloe vera gel juice). Swish for a few minutes and spit. Do this twice a day. Do not swallow this mixture.

When dealing with issues in your mouth, make sure you also work to fix the root cause, which is usually related to digestion and diet, especially vitamin and mineral deficiencies. I also suggest brushing with a remineralizing toothpaste. I make a product called Dubh Toothsoap, which contains all the necessary minerals. It can also be a good idea to add boron, magnesium, and vitamin K2 supplements to any bone- or tooth-healing regime.

Scalp Care and Hair Growth Formula

100 mL glass spray bottle	30 mL distilled water
50 mL 99.995 percent pharmaceutical-grade DMSO	6 drops 100 percent pure essential oil of rosemary
20 mL preservative-free aloe vera gel juice	4 drops 100 percent pure essential oil of peppermint

Since formulating my DMSO hair growth spray, I have had many happy testimonials about how the spray helped not only grow hair but also heal the scalp, put an end to dandruff, balance oils, and reduce gray hairs. I infuse the solution I sell in my store with horsetail (*Equisetum arvense*), also called bottlebrush or shavegrass, and add rosemary and peppermint extracts as well, but here's a simpler solution that you can easily make at home.

Using a funnel, pour the DMSO into the glass spray bottle. Add the aloe vera gel juice, distilled water, and essential oils of rosemary and peppermint. Replace the spray nozzle and shake well. Spray on clean, dry hair and scalp. Make sure you use all-natural shampoo and conditioner to clean your hair. Use as many sprays as needed to cover the target area in a larger circumference than the area you are trying to treat. Let the spray absorb fully. Shake the bottle well in between applications. For long-standing alopecia or male pattern baldness, be consistent with applications; one to two times daily is ideal. In some cases, it can take up to a year of use to see serious growth.

Topical Vitamin and Mineral Blend

50 mL glass dropper bottle

1 mL magnesium oil

2 drops Lugol's iodine
or povidone-iodine

powder from ½
capsule vitamin C

powder from ½ capsule
B-complex vitamin

40 mL 99.995 percent
pharmaceutical-grade DMSO

10 mL preservative-free
aloe vera gel juice

Place a funnel over the glass dropper bottle. Add the magnesium oil, iodine, C and B-complex vitamins, DMSO, and aloe vera gel juice. Shake well. Store in a cool, dark place and make a new mixture after six months. This blend is for topical use only. Apply 3 to 5 mL of solution on any area of the body you are trying to heal one or two times a day. Once you are comfortable using this blend, you can experiment with adding different vitamins or minerals to new blends.

Conclusion

Hopefully you will find the above recipes useful for your at-home remedies. If you are interested in exploring other homeopathic and naturopathic home remedies, feel free to explore my website yummy-mummyemporium.ca. As I've stated before, it is important to consult with your doctor or a medical professional before implementing any of these blends, sprays, and drops into your health regimen. Your health is top priority!

CHAPTER 7

How to Use DMSO for Our Animal Friends

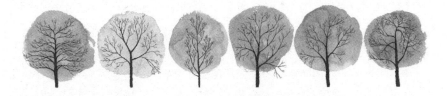

My original training was in veterinary medicine, as my undergraduate science degree reflects, and I did many years of paid and volunteer work in various vet clinics, zoos, and wildlife centers. As well, my parents rescued feral cats, taking responsibility for a very large cat colony in my hometown. The township, Humane Society, and local citizens ignored this growing problem, so there were always animals around me in need of care. I was also blessed to work in a holistic veterinary clinic that beautifully blended conventional veterinary approaches and naturopathic principles. It was here that I learned about the power of homeopathy and traditional Chinese medicine. Being able to taste and sample the impressive array of botanical medicines the doctors had in the clinic and witnessing the miraculous effects of acupuncture on animals molded me into the medicine woman I am today. Then I took distance courses in animal homeopathy from the British Institute of Homeopathy to learn more. I was thrilled when I made the top 100 accepted for an interview at the University of Guelph, a school well known for its veterinary program. However, they were unimpressed that I had such a passion for holistic vet medicine and I was turned down, quite aggressively so. I decided to pursue other learning venues, knowing I could still use the information to help animals whenever I could.

Over the past 20 years, I've used a plethora of natural remedies on animals. They include homeopathics, colloidal silver, certain herbal remedies, dietary changes, water changes, and now, of course, DMSO.

There is a long history of DMSO use on horses, but for this book I am focusing on our small animal friends like cats and dogs. DMSO is safe for use in dogs and has been FDA approved for treating musculoskeletal disorders. It is excellent for helping with joint pain, swelling, inflammation, and even scleroderma and lupus. DMSO can be used on any mammal or reptile, but the responsibility of the dose is up to you. Rules for animals: Keep the doses low, always test a small patch first to check for sensitivity, and at any sign of a negative reaction, discontinue use and consult a qualified practitioner or veterinarian.

DMSO Dosing for Pets

When using DMSO on animals, it's important to take age and weight into consideration. Use between one eighth and one quarter of the human dose in general. My rule of thumb is 2 ml of pure DMSO for every 10 pounds of body weight in enough distilled water to dilute it between 20 and 50 percent, for internal application. It can be added into food or syringed into the mouth. For topical application, apply 2 ml pure DMSO in 2 ml of distilled water (making a 50 percent solution) and apply it on areas where there is less fur (ears, nose, belly, paws), or rub it into the fur. I have used 90 percent DMSO on surgical wounds, but when using higher doses it's best to work with a holistic practitioner who has experience treating animals with DMSO.

Infections and Injuries

Clean the affected area with warm water, then cleanse with colloidal silver. You can also use rubbing alcohol as a cleanser and to help reduce swelling. Apply a 50 percent DMSO solution that was diluted with distilled water or colloidal silver to the affected area. Always give homeopathic *Arnica montana* 30CH or whatever potency you have on hand in case of injury, especially with bleeding and bruising. Dilute 3 pellets in a little distilled water and give a 30CH dose three to six times a day via clean syringe.

Eyes

You can use the 20 percent DMSO eye drops (see page 96) to treat an animal's cataracts. It is a good idea to make plain, normal saline to soothe the animal's eyes after using the DMSO eye drops; animals can be much more sensitive to DMSO than humans. If the animal doesn't tolerate the 20 percent solution, then make a 10 percent solution instead. You can buy these solutions on the internet, some have added vitamin C or glutathione, which are safe to use, just be aware than they will sting slightly more with nutrients included than without.

Chronic Disease Approach

For treatment of symptoms of cancers, organ problems, and seizures, give 7 to 10 drops of pure DMSO in at least the same amount (and up to 1 ounce) of distilled water or preservative-free aloe vera gel juice in the mouth with a syringe once or twice a day. This is the dose for a medium-weight cat or a small dog. More or less will need to be used depending on the animal's weight as per the ratio I have already mentioned. You also need to apply DMSO topically, change the diet, and target the specific organs that need detoxing and balance, so it's crucial to work with a qualified holistic veterinarian or practitioner who knows how to guide the case.

Conclusion

There are a variety of effective natural remedies that can be used on pets, but there is enough information on that subject to fill an entirely new book! If you are curious about other naturopathic or homeopathic remedies for your pets, I recommend the following books: *The Complete Herbal Handbook for the Dog and Cat* by Juliette de Baïracli Levy (affectionately known as Juliette of the Herbs), *The Encyclopedia of Natural Pet Care* by CJ Puotinen, *The Homeopathic Treatment of Small Animals* by Christopher Day, and *A Veterinary Materia Medica and Clinical Repertory* by George MacLeod. These are the books I consult time and time again.

CHAPTER 8

FDA-Approved Medical Usages of DMSO

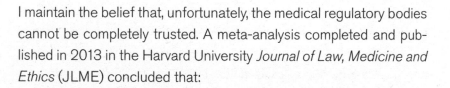

I maintain the belief that, unfortunately, the medical regulatory bodies cannot be completely trusted. A meta-analysis completed and published in 2013 in the Harvard University *Journal of Law, Medicine and Ethics* (JLME) concluded that:

- 90% of FDA-approved drugs provide no better treatment than existing drugs (over a 30-year study span).

- Prescription drugs are the fourth leading cause of death in America and Americans experience over 80 million drug side effects that can be life debilitating.

- There is evidence that since the pharmaceutical industry started making large contributions to the FDA for reviewing drugs and has paid congressmen to accept private funding rather than using public oversight, this has led the FDA to speed up the drug review process, further endangering the American public.

- The FDA legitimizes the marketing ploy "the selling of sickness" to invent new categories of illness for which drugs can then be prescribed for.
- Convenient regulations exist preventing the FDA from price comparing similar drugs or testing their cost effectiveness.
- Only in the U.S. are drug companies allowed, without restriction, to sell their drugs for however much they like and continue to raise the prices year after year.[94]

With the thousands of DMSO studies and loads of clinical evidence of the safety and profound health benefits dimethyl sulfoxide provides, these agencies should have long since embraced this substance, shared the information at length with both doctors and the public, and funded further agencies to promote the creation of DMSO-containing products. However, here we are in a world where most of the population and most doctors have never even heard of it.

DMSO has been embraced by the pharmaceutical industry as a drug delivery agent, however, so the FDA has approved it for their usage. For anyone with a scientific mind who is interested in delving deeper into this handful of approved medical uses of DMSO, here are some interesting treatments, solutions, and other applications, again high-lighting the wide range and versatility of DMSO.

RIMSO

One of the earliest parenteral (meaning something that is not admin-istered via the gastrointestinal tract) products approved in the United States is RIMSO-50. It is a 50 percent sterile, non-heat causing, watery DMSO formulation used to help manage the symptoms of interstitial cystitis, a condition of the bladder wall.[95] RIMSO-50 is slowly instilled into a patient's bladder using a catheter or a syringe and remains in the bladder for 10 to 15 minutes. DMSO has long been used to treat interstitial cystitis and is considered very safe, with no long-term side effects.[96, 97]

Approved Devices

The following are FDA-approved devices containing or using DMSO in some manner and that are currently available through a medical doctor. I include this information for two reasons: to help you understand that the medical industry is aware of the value of DMSO and its use in many conventional applications, and to make you aware of these applications so you can mention them to your doctor if you have a related condition.

- **Onyx** is medical polymer in a DMSO solution, which is injected into the bloodstream to treat intracranial aneurysms. The technical name for this device is liquid embolic system. Once injected, the DMSO dissolves, leaving a glue-like material that fills the aneurysm space, solidifies into a spongy material, and prevents the aneurysm from rupturing. Onyx is made by Microtherapeutics Corporation of Irvine, California.

(Side note: I would design an injectable remedy of homeopathic *Arnica montana* and/or yarrow dissolved in DMSO to treat this condition; these botanical plants are two of the best remedies to halt bleeding as well as assist in tissue regeneration.)

- **Tegress** is somewhat similar to Onyx; it serves as a bulking agent inside the urethra and also uses DMSO as a carrier.[98] Tegress is made by C. R. Bard in New Jersey.

- **Viadur** is another device that uses DMSO as a solubilizing excipient (meaning it dissolves and carries the drug), as a drug delivery agent for the treatment of prostate cancer.[99] This 12-month treatment, in which the device is implanted in the upper arm, slowly releases a solution of DMSO (104 mg) and leuprolide acetate (72 mg). The manufacturer is Bayer Healthcare Pharmaceuticals in Germany.

Transdermal

Many agents are transdermal, some absorbing rapidly and others only after a lengthy stay. Many toxins are also able to penetrate the skin's layers. It is therefore crucial to understand how important it is not to smother our skin with toxic chemicals that are readily found in many cosmetics and topical products. As well, keeping our skin clean and breathable is equally as important, as it is a two-way street. For more information on this, I recommend that you research the topic gua sha. The following list is included for you to use as a reference guide when shopping for cosmetics, so you can steer clear of chemicals that can damage your health.

A summary of the permeation enhancers used in the transdermal industry, organized from most toxicity to least (or null) toxicity:

- Surfactants (sodium laureate, cetyltrimethylammonium bromide, Brij®, Tween®, and sodium cholate),
- Hydrocarbons (alkanes and squalene),
- Alcohols (ethanol, pentanol, benzyl alcohol, lauryl alcohol, propylene glycols, and glycerol),
- Amides (1-dodecylazacycloheptane-2-one [Azone®], urea, dimethylacetamide, dimethylformamide, and pyrrolidone derivatives),

- Amines (diethanolamine and triethanolamine),
- Fatty acids (oleic acid, linoleic acid, valeric acid, and lauric acid),
- Esters (isopropyl palmitate, isopropyl myristate, and ethyl acetate),
- Terpenes (D-limonene, carvone, and anise oil),
- Phospholipids (lecithin), and
- Sulfoxides (dimethyl sulfoxide).[100, 101, 102]

These various chemical groups represent substances which have the ability to cross the skin layers and move into the bloodstream. About half of this list are toxic to the body while the others are safe. And of the items in the list, DMSO has by far the most transdermal, healing, and carrying capacity.

Cryopreservation

DMSO has long been used to preserve bone marrow and blood components at low temperatures. DMSO is "generally acceptable" as a cryoprotectant for use in human cells, tissues, and cellular and tissue-based products (HCT/Ps), as defined by the FDA.[103, 104]

In the United States, pharmaceutical-grade DMSO is widely used for the cryopreservation of stem cells from umbilical cord blood at childbirth. Cord blood is injected to treat certain human disorders that affect the blood and immune system, such as genetic disorders.

Products for Animal Health Approved in the United States

DMSO for use in horses is well established, and most horse breeders are aware of its variety of applications. Domoso, a 90 percent

DMSO solution available in both liquid and gel formations, is indicated for acute swelling in horses.[105] Most equine groups have used DMSO long enough to be aware of its value as an off-label product (meaning used for a condition for which it has not been officially approved). Top health issues diagnosed in horses include musculoskeletal injuries, arthritis, and joint disease. DMSO is often used by caregivers to ease pain and inflammation caused by these common issues, and to encourage healing. Feeding tubes are frequently used to deliver DMSO into the stomach or intestines of horses. In horse racing, where drug-testing regulations are very specific, it's important to know that DMSO can concentrate certain drugs.

Synotic, which contains 60 percent DMSO, is used by veterinarians to treat ear infections in dogs.

DMSO-Containing Products Marketed outside the United States

The antiviral idoxuridine is used for the treatment of shingles in Europe.[106] DMSO is used with the idoxuridine in penetrating the tissues and reaching the damaged cells.

In Canada and the European Union, there are DMSO-containing topical products for the treatment of certain types of joint pain. Dolicur (Schering AG) is an approved DMSO product in Germany, as an over-the-counter treatment for sports-related injuries, and laws exist in various Russian provinces that allow for DMSO self-medication.[107] In China, DMSO is also widely used as a topical remedy for self-medicated topical pain relief.

Other Names Used for DMSO

There are various names for DMSO and in a variety of languages. Many of the English names include dimethyl sulfoxide (two words), dimethylsulfoxide (one word), dimethyl sulphoxide, methyl sulphoxide, Me2SO, NSC-763, SQ-9453, and sulphinybismethane. This is helpful if you are interested in researching further, as you may not find certain studies using just the key words DMSO or dimethyl sulfoxide.

Conclusion

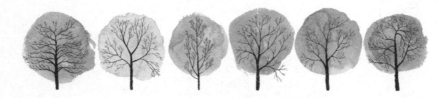

It has been my every intention to assist you, dear reader, upon finishing this book, in carrying a new level of knowledge, a new skill, and a newfound freedom: the empowerment of knowing about DMSO and how to use it well. Within you now is an awareness that so few yet possess, and on your shelf, a guidebook that can help you navigate, with confidence, common ailments that we so often face in life.

It is my every desire to see humanity flourish, rise in health, overcome injustice, expose corruption, and live in a peaceful coexistence with nature. As we share knowledge, we learn better self-care and take self-responsibility for our own health, preventing disease before it strikes and listening to the signs our bodies give us so we know we need to change our habits. When we heal, we can carry more energy and care for others, working together to solve problems and build a world filled with love and kindness. It is our birthright and it is up to us to claim it.

Please share this book with others. Tell them about it. Ask them if they have ever heard about DMSO. Remind them how our Creator made all that we need for our peace, health, and happiness in the plants that grow all around us. Let them know there is another way to feel better, that there is hope for their well-being, that there is a better way.

I thank you for reading my words, for understanding my passion for natural health, and for taking the time to learn about DMSO. The wisdom of the trees now walks with you. May you walk well.

Endnotes

1   Irena Kratochvílová et al., "Theoretical and Experimental Study of the Antifreeze Protein AFP752, Trehalose and Dimethyl Sulfoxide Cryoprotection Mechanism: Correlation with Cryopreserved Cell Viability," *RCS Advances* 7, no. 1 (2017): 352–60.

2   Patrick McGrady Sr., *The Persecuted Drug: The Story of DMSO* (New York: Charter Books, 1980).

3   Chauncey D. Leake et al., "Biological Actions of Dimethyl Sulfoxide," *Annals of the New York Academy of Sciences* 243, no. 1 (1967): 5–508.

4   Hagens Berman, "Number of Thalidomide Victims in US Vastly Underreported, Lawsuit Claims," last modified October 25, 2011, https://www.hbsslaw.com/cases/thalidomide/pressrelease/thalidomide-number-of-thalidomide-victims-in-us-vastly-underreported-lawsuit-claims.

5   Stanley W. Jacob, interview by Mike Wallace, "The Riddle of DMSO," *Sixty Minutes,* CBS, March 23, 1980.

6   Stanley W. Jacob, interview by Mike Wallace, "The Riddle of DMS."

7   Elizabeth C. Asher et al., "Measurement of DMS, DMSO, and DMSP in Natural Waters by Automated Sequential Chemical Analysis," *Methods* 13, no. 9 (2015): 451–62, doi: 10.1002/lom3.10039.

8   Stanley W. Jacob and Jack C. de la Torre, *Dimethyl Sulfoxide (DMSO) in Trauma and Disease* (Boca Raton, FL: CRC Press, 2015).

9   Poornima Tamma, "Organ Transport Could Get Chillier with New UT Research," *The Daily Texan,* July 13, 2017, http://www.dailytexanonline.com/2017/07/13/organ-transport-could-get-chillier-with-new-ut-research.

10   Rebecca Notman et al., "The Permeability Enhancing Mechanism of DMSO in Ceramide Bilayers Simulated by Molecular Dynamics," *Biophysical Journal* 93, no. 6 (2007): 2056–68, doi: 10.1529/biophysj.107.104703.

11   T. C. Moore et al., "The Influence of Ceramide Tail Length on the Structure of Bilayers Composed of Stratum Corneum Lipids," *Biophysical Journal* 114 (2018): 113–25.

12   Gabriela Segura, "DMSO: The Real Miracle Solution," last modified May 12, 2011, https://www.sott.net/article/228453-DMSO-The-Real-Miracle-Solution.

13   Hartmut Fischer and Seiriol Dafydd, *The DMSO Handbook: A New Paradigm in Healthcare* (Schnaittach: Daniel Peter Verlag, 2015).

14   Masami Noda et al., "A Single-Molecule Assessment of the Protective Effect of DMSO Against DNA Double-Strand Breaks Induced by Photo-and Y-Ray-Irradiation, and Freezing," *Scientific Reports* 7 (August 2017): 8557, doi:10.1038/s41598-017-08894-y.

15   Thomas W. Pearson, Howard J. Dawson, and Homer B. Lackey, "Naturally Occurring Levels of Dimethyl Sulfoxide in Selected Fruits, Vegetables, Grains, and Beverages," *Journal of Agriculture and Food Chemistry* 29, no. 5 (1981): 1089–91, doi:10.1021/jf00107a049.

16   De Pinieux et al., "Lipid-Lowering Drugs and Mitochondrial Function: Effects of HMG-CoA Reductase Inhibitors on Serum Ubiquinone and Blood Lactate/Pyruvate Ratio," *British Journal of Clinical Pharmacology* 42, no. 3 (September 1996): 333-37, doi: 10.1046/j.1365-2125.1996.04178.x

17   E. G. Bliznakov EG and D. J. Wilkins, "Biochemical and Clinical Consequences of Inhibiting Coenzyme Q10 Biosynthesis by Lipid-Lowering HMG-CoA Reductase Inhibitors (Statins). A Critical Review," *Advances in Therapy* 15, no. 4 (July 1998): 218–28.

18   "Whitaker J. Citizens' Petition Filed with FDA to Include Coenzyme Q10 Use Recommendation in All Statin Drug Labelling," *Life Extension Magazine*, May 23, 2002.

19   Karl Folkers et al., "Lovastatin Decreases Coenzyme Q Levels in Humans," *Proceedings of the National Academy of Sciences* 87, no. 22 (November 1990): 8931–34, doi: 10.1073/pnas.87.22.8931.

20   Umme Aiman, Ahmad Najmi, and Rahat Ali Khan, "Statin Induced Diabetes and Its Clinical Implications," *Journal of Pharmacology and Pharmacotherapeutics* 5, no. 3 (2014): 181–85, doi: 10.4103/0976-500X.136097.

21   Justin Smith, *$29 Billion Reasons to Lie about Cholesterol: Making Profit by Turning Healthy People into Patients* (Leicester, England: Matador, 2009).

22   Patrick McGrady, *The Persecuted Drug* (New York: Charter Communication, 1980), 58–59.

23   Andrey A. Gurtovenko and Jamshed Anwar, "Modulating the Structure and Properties of Cell Membranes: The Molecular Mechanism of Action of Dimethyl Sulfoxide," *The Journal of Physical Chemistry* 111, no. 35 (2007): 10453–60, doi: 10.1021/jp073113e.

24   R. A. Aubin, et al., "Polybrene/DMSO-Assisted Gene Transfer," *Molecular Biotechnology* 1, no. 1 (1994): 29-48. 10.1007/BF02821509.

25   Lyra Nara, "Nature's Best Healer," accessed November 19, 2019, https://lyranara.me/dmso.

26   K. Formanek and W. Kovak, "Die Wirkung Von DMSO Auf Experimentell Erzeugte Rattenpfotenodeme, in *DMSO Symposium*, Vienna, Austria. Saladruk, Berlin, Germany, 1966: 18–26.

27   P. Gorog and I. B. Kovacs, "Effect of Dimethyl Sulfoxide (DMSO) on Various Experimental Inflammations," *Current Therapuetic Reasearch* 10, no. 9 (1968): 486–92.

28   Stanley Jacob and Jack C. De La Torre, *Dimethyl Sulfoxide in Trauma and Disease* (Boca Raton, FL: CRC Press, 2015).

29   M. Johnson and P. W. Ramwell, *Implications of Prostaglandins in Hematology* (New York: Academic Press, 1974), 275–304.

30   P. B. Weiser, M. A. Zeiger, and J. N. Falin, "Effects on Dimethyl Sulfoxide on Cyclic AMP Accumulation, Lipolysis and Glucose Metabolism of Fat Cells," *Biochemical Pharmacology* 26, no. 8 (1977): 775–78.

31   P. Gorog and I. B. Kovacs, "Effect of Dimethyl Sulfoxide (DMSO) on Various Experimental Cutaneous Reactions," *Pharmacology* 2, no. 5 (1969): 313–19, doi: 10.1159/000136034.

32   G. Weissmann, G. Sessa, and V. Bevans, "Effect of DMSO on the Stabilization of Lysosomes by Cortisone and Chloroquine in Vitro," *Annals of the New York Academy of Sciences* 141, no. 1 (1967): 326–32.

33   W. M. Sams Jr., "The Effects of Dimethyl Sulfoxide on Nerve Conduction," *Annals of the New York Academy of Sciences* 141, no. 1 (1967): 242–47.

34   C. Norman Shealy, "The Physiological Substrate of Pain," *Headache: The Journal of Head and Face Pain* 6, no. 3 (1966): 101–8.

35   Anu Rahal et al., "Oxidative Stress, Prooxidants, and Antioxidants: The Inter-play," *BioMed Research International* (2014): 761264, doi:10.1155/2014/761264.

36   Ronald Houwing et al., "An Unexpected Detrimental Effect on the Incidence of Heel Pressure Ulcers after Local 5% DMSO Cream Application: A Randomized, Double-blind Study in Patients at Risk for Pressure Ulcers," *Wounds* 20, no. 4 (2008): 84-8.

37   Houwing et al., "An Unexpected Detrimental Effect."

38   Y. Wu, Z. Huang, Y. Luo et al., "X-ray Absorption and Electron Paramagnetic Resonance Guided Discovery of the Cu-Catalyzed Synthesis of Multiaryl-Substituted Furans from Aryl Styrene and Ketones Using DMSO as the Oxidant," *Organic Letters* 19, no. 9 (2017): 2330–33.

39   Harry H. Szmant, "Physical Properties of Dimethyl Sulfoxide and Its Function in Biological Systems," *Annals of the New York Academy of Sciences* 243, no. 1 (1975): 20–23.

40   Carolina Sanmartin-Suarez, "Antioxidant Properties of Dimethyl Sulfoxide and Its Viability as a Solvent in the Evaluation of Neuroprotective Antioxidants," *Journal of Pharmacological and Toxicological Method* 63, no. 2 (2010): 209–15.

41   Jacob and De La Torre, *Dimethyl Sulfoxide in Trauma and Disease.*

42   R. D. Broadwell, M. Salcman, and R. S. Kaplan, "Morphologic Effect of Dimethyl Sulfoxide on the Blood–Brain Barrier," *Science* 217, no. 4555 (1982):164–66, doi :10.1126/science/7089551.

43   Jacob and De La Torre, *Dimethyl Sulfoxide in Trauma and Disease.*

44   Genro Kashino, Yong Liu, Minoru Suzuki, Shin-ichiro Masunaga, Yuko Kinashi, Koja Ono, Keiz Tano, and Masami Watanabe. "An Alternative Mechanism for Radioprotection by Dimethyl Sulfoxide, Possible Facilitation of DNA Double Strand Break Repair," *Journal of Radiation Research*, 51 no. 6 (2010): 733–40, doi: 10.1269/jrr.09106.

45   Glenn E. Pottz, James H. Rampey, and Furmandean Benjamin, "The Effect of Dimethyl Sulfoxide (DMSO) on Antibiotic Sensitivity of a Group of Medically Important Microorganisms: Preliminary Report," *Annals of the New York Academy of Sciences* 141, no. 1 (1967): 261–72, doi: 10.1111/j.1749-6632.1967.tb34888.x.

46   H. Basch and H. H. Gadebusch, "In Vitro Antimicrobial Activity of Dimethylsulfoxide," *Applied Microbiology* 16, no. 12 (1968): 1953–54.

47   Jacob and De La Torre, *Dimethyl Sulfoxide in Trauma and Disease.*

48   T. Szydlowska and I. Pawloska, "In Vivo Studies on Reversion to Sensitivity of INH-resistant Tubercle Bacilli under the Influence of Dimethylsulfoxide (DMSO)," *Archivum Immunologiae Therapiae Experimentalis* 22, no. 4 (1974): 559–61.

49   R. D. Broadwell, M. Salcman, and R. S. Kaplan, "Morphologic Effect of Dimethyl Sulfoxide on the Blood–Brain Barrier," *Science* 217, no. 4555 (1982):164–66, doi :10.1126/science/7089551.

50   G. B. Bradham and J. J. Sample. "The Vascular and Thermal Effects of Dimethyl Sulfoxide," *Annals of New York Academy of Sciences* 141 no. 1 (March 1967): 225–30, doi: 10.1111/j.1749-6632.1967.tb34883.x.

51   S. Rehncrona, B. K. Siesjo, and D. S. Smith, "Reversible Ischemia of the Brain: Biochemical Factors Influencing Restitution," *Acta Physiologia Scandinavica Supplementum* 492 (1980): 135–40.

52   T. Kaneda, et al., "Endothelium Dependent and Independent Vasodilator Effects of Dimethyl Sulfoxide in Rat Aorta," *Pharmacology* 97, no. 3–4 (2016): 171-76, doi: 10.1159/000443894.

53   I. G. P. Duimel-Peeters et al., "A Systematic Review of the Efficacy of Topical Skin Application of Dimethyl Sulfoxide on Wound Healing and as an Anti-Inflammatory," *Wounds* 15, no. 12 (2003): 361–70.

54   N. C. Santos et al., "Multidisciplinary Utilization of Dimethyl Sulfoxide: Pharmacological, Cellular, and Molecular Aspects," *Biochemical Pharmacology* 65, no. 7 (2003): 1035–41.

55   M. Muir, "DMSO: Many Uses, Much Controversy," *Alternative and Complementary Therapies* 2 (July/August 1996): 230–235.

56   Y. Tachi, Y. Okuda, C. Bannai, N. Okamura, S. Bannai, K. Yamashita. "High Concentration of Glucose Causes Impairment of the Function of the Glutathione Redox Cycle in Human Vascular Smooth Muscle Cells," *FEBS Letters* 421 no. 1 (1998): 19–22, doi: 10.1016/s0014-5793(97)01526-3.

57   Jeanne A. Drisko, "Chelation Therapy" in *Integrative Medicine,* ed. David Rakel (Amsterdam: Elsevier, 2017), 1004–15.

58   Archie H. Scott, *The DMSO Handbook for Doctors* (Bloomington, IL: iUniverse, 2013).

59   Jennifer L. Hanslick et al., "Dimethyl Sulfoxide (DMSO) Produces Widespread Apoptosis in the Developing Central Nervous System," *Neurobiology of Disease* 34, no. 1 (2009): 1–10.

60 M. A. Higman et al., "Reversible Leukoencephalopathy Associated with Re-infusion of DMSO Preserved Stem Cells," *Bone Marrow Transplant* 26, no. 7 (2000): 797–800.

61 H. J. Mallach, "Interaction of DMSO and Alcohol," *Annals of the New York Academy of Sciences* 141, no. 1 (1967): 457–62.

62 Lee S. Simona et al., "Efficacy and Safety of Topical Diclofenac Containing Dimethyl Sulfoxide (DMSO) Compared with Those of Topical Placebo, DMSO Vehicle and Oral Diclofenac for Knee Osteoarthritis," *Pain* 143, no. 3 (2009): 238–45.

63 Robert L. Perlman and J. Wolff, "Dimethyl Sulfoxide: An Inhibitor of Liver Alcohol Dehydrogenase," *Science* 160, no. 3825 (1968): 317–19.

64 Heather Smith Thomas, "Harnessing the Power of DMSO," Equus, last modified March 10, 2017, https://equusmagazine.com/lameness/dmso-for-horses-8468.

65 P. A. Doig, "Dimethyl Sulfoxide and Alcohol—A Potentially Dangerous Combination," *Canadian Veterinary Journal* 40, no. 11 (1999): 755–56.

66 Jessamine Ng Lee, Cheolmin Park, and George M. Whitesides, "Solvent Compatibility of Poly(dimethylsiloxane)-Based Microfluidic Devices," *Analytical Chemistry* 75, no. 23 (2003): 6544–54.

67 Heal Yourself at Home, "DMSO Compatibility with Plastics Types and Other Materials," accessed November 20, 2019, http://healyourselfathome.com/HOW/THERAPIES/DMSO-MSM/DMSO_compatibility_chart.aspx.

68 Heal Yourself at Home, "DMSO Compatibility with Plastics."

69 Rene Miranda-Tirado, "Dimethyl Sulfoxide Therapy in Chronic Skin Ulcers," *Annals of the New York Academy of Sciences* 243 (1975): 408–11.

70 Alison Vickery, "Natural Antihistamine," December 21, 2013, https://alisonvickery.com.au/natural-antihistamine.

71 Ayman Atiba and Alaa Ghazy, "The Effects of Topical Dimethyle Sulfoxide on Second-Degree Burn Wound Healing in Dogs," *Alexandria Journal of Veterinary Sciences* 45 (2015): 6–12.

72 S. Shimizu, R. P. Simon, and S. H. Graham, "Dimethylsulfoxide (DMSO) Treatment Reduces Infarction Volume after Focal Cerebral Ischemia in Rats," *Neuroscience Letter* 239, no. 2–3 (1997): 125–27.

73   H. Baschand and H. H. Gadebusch, "In Vitro Antimicrobial Activity of Dimethylsulfoxide," *Applied Microbiology* 16, no. 12 (1968): 1953–54.

74   Archie H. Scott, *The DMSO Handbook for Doctors* (Bloomington, IL: iUniverse, 2013).

75   John Heinz and Laudahn Gerhard, "Clinical Experiences with the Topical Application of DMSO in Orthopedic Diseases: Evaluation of 4180 Cases," *Annals of the New York Academy of Science* 141, no. 1 (1967): 506–16.

76   M. Gaspar et al., "Efficacy of a Topical Treatment Protocol with Dimethyl Sulfoxide 50% in Type 1 Complex Regional Pain Syndrome," *Farmacia Hospitilaria* 36, no. 5 (2012): 385–91.

77   "Vitamins B6 And B12 Could Relieve Painful Carpal Tunnel Symptoms," Dr. Glenn S. Rothfield's Nutrition and Healing, accessed November 20, 2019, https://nutritionandhealing.com/2013/07/29/vitamins-b6-and-b12.

78   E. C. Percy and J. D. Carson, "The Use of DMSO in Tennis Elbow and Rotator Cuff Tendonitis: A Double-Blind Study," *Medicine and Science in Sports and Exercise* 13, no. 4 (1981): 215–19.

79   J. H. Brown, "Clinical Experience with DMSO in Acute Musculoskeletal Conditions Comparing a Noncontrolled Series with a Controlled Double Blind Study," *Annals of the New York Academy of Sciences* 141, no. 1 (1967): 496–505.

80   A. Steinberg, "The Employment of Dimethyl Sulfoxide as an Anti-Inflammatory Agent and Steroid-Transporter in Diversified Clinical Disease," *Annals of the New York Academy of Sciences* 141, no. 1 (1967): 532–50.

81   Jacob and De La Torre, *Dimethyl Sulfoxide in Trauma and Disease.*

82   Jacob and De La Torre, *Dimethyl Sulfoxide in Trauma and Disease.*

83   Michael E. Benros et al., "Autoimmune Diseases and Severe Infections as Risk Factors for Mood Disorders: A Nationwide Study," *JAMA Psychiatry* 70, no. 8 (2013): 812–20.

84   Johann Steiner et al., "Severe Depression Is Associated with Increased Microglial Quinolinic Acid in Subregions of the Anterior Cingulate Gyrus: Evidence for an Immune-Modulated Glutamatergic Neurotransmission?" *Journal of Neuroinflammation* 8, no. 94 (August 2011): doi:10.1186/1742-2094-8-94.

85   Elaine Setiawan et al., "Role of Translocator Protein Density, a Marker of Neuroinflammation, in the Brain during Major Depressive Episodes," *JAMA Psychiatry* 72, no. 3 (2015): 268–75, doi:10.1001/jamapsychiatry.2014.2427.

86   Elaine Setiawan et al., "Association of Translocator Protein Total Distribution Volume with Duration of Untreated Major Depressive Disorder: A Cross-Sectional Study," *The Lancet* 5, no. 4 (2018): 339–47.

87   Eduardo Ramirez and Segisfredo Luza, "Dimethyl Sulfoxide in the Treatment of Mental Patients," *Annals of the New York Academy of Sciences* 141, no. 1 (1967): 655–67.

88   Ramirez and Luza, "Dimethyl Sulfoxide in the Treatment of Mental Patients," 655–67.

89   D. M. Gordon and K. E. Kleberger. "The Effect of Dimethyl Sulfoxide (DMSO) on Animal and Human Eyes," *Archives of Ophthalmology* 79, no. 4 (1968): 423–27.

90   Jun Matsumoto, "Clinical Trials of Dimethyl Sulfoxide in Rheumatoid Arthritis Patients in Japan," *Annals of the New York Academy of Sciences* 141, no. 1 (1967): 560–68.

91   Castor Oil, "Undecylenic Acid," last modified 2018, http://www.castoroil.in/castor/castor_seed/castor_oil/c11/undecylenic_acid/undecylenic_acid.html.

92   J. M. Caron et al., "Methyl Sulfone Induces Loss of Metastatic Properties and Reemergence of Normal Phenotypes in a Metastatic Cloudman S-91 (M3) Murine Melanoma Cell Line," *PloS One* 5 no. 8 (August 2010): e11788, doi:10.1371/journal.pone.0011788.

93   Tony St. Leger, "Meet the Eye Microbiome," *Scientific American,* June 23, 2019, https://www.scientificamerican.com/article/meet-the-eye-microbiome/.

94   Donald W. Light, Joel Lexchin, and Jonathan J. Darrow, "Institutional Corruption of Pharmaceuticals and the Myth of Safe and Effective Drugs," *Journal of Law, Medicine and Ethics* 14, no. 3 (June 1, 2013): 590–610, https://ssrn.com/abstract=2282014.

95   A.M.A. Department of Drugs, *Agents Used to Treat Interstitial Cystitis in A.M.A. Drug Evaluations* (Chicago: American Medical Association, 1980), 617–18.

96   S. W. Shirley, B. H. Stewart, and S. Mirelman, "Dimethyl Sulfoxide in Treatment of Inflammatory Genitourinary Disorders," *Urology* 11, no. 3 (1978): 215–20.

97   J. Rössberger, M. Fall, and R. Peeker, "Critical Appraisal of Dimethyl Sulfoxide Treatment for Interstitial Cystitis: Discomfort, Side-Effects and Treatment Outcome," *Scandinavian Journal of Urology and Nephrology* 39, no. 1 (2005): 73–77.

98   Roger R. Dmochowski, "Tegress Urethral Implant Phase III Clinical Experience and Product Uniqueness," *Reviews in Urology* 7 (2005): S22–S26.

99   R. G. Strickley, "Solubilizing Excipients in Oral and Injectable Formulations," *Pharmaceutical Research* 21, no. 2 (2004): 201–30.

100   Kalpana S. Paudel et al., "Challenges and Opportunities in Dermal/ Transdermal Delivery," *Therapeutic Delivery* 1, no. 1 (2011): 109–31.

101   D. Prabhakar, J. Sreekanth, and K. N. Jayaveera, "Effect of Dimethylsulfoxide on Transdermal Patches of Azelnidipine, "*Der Pharmacia Lettre* 6, no. 1 (2014): 120–27.

102   U.S. Food and Drug Administration, "Fentanyl Transdermal System (Marketed as Duragesic) Information," July 10, 2015, https://www.fda.gov/drugs/ postmarket-drug-safety-information-patients-and-providers/fentanyl-transdermal-system-marketed-duragesic-information.

103   U.S. Food and Drug Administration, "Code of Federal Regulations Title," 21, April 1, 2018, https://www.accessdata.fda.gov/scripts/cdrh/cfdocs/cfCFR/ CFRSearch.cfm.

104   U.S. Food and Drug Administration, "NucliSens HIV-1 QT," last modified November 13, 2001, https://www.fda.gov/media/73107/download.

105   C. F. Brayton,"Dimethyl Sulfoxide (DMSO): A Review," *Cornell Veterinarian* 76, no. 1 (1986): 61–90.

106   A. Aliaga et al., "A Topical Solution of 40% Idoxuridine in Dimethyl Sulfoxide Compared to Oral Acyclovir in the Treatment of Herpes Zoster. A Double-Blind Multicenter Clinical Trial," *Medicina Clínica* 98, no. 7 (1992): 245–49.

107   Alexandra Ely and B. Lockwood, "What Is the Evidence for the Safety and Efficacy of Dimethyl Sulfoxide and Methylsulfonylmethane in Pain Relief?," *Pharmaceutical Journal* 269, no. 7223 (2002): 685–87.

Index

industrial grade, 13–14
   pharmaceutical grade, 14
Graham, S. H., 121n72
Gurtovenko, Andrey A., 118n23

H

hair growth, 75, 101
Hanslick, Jennifer L., 120n59
headaches, 59–60
head trauma, 66–67
healing burns, 57
healing crisis, 16–17, 35
healing substances, 18
Heinz, John, 122n75
hemorrhagic stroke, 29
hemorrhoids, 76–77
Herxheimer reaction, 17
high-density polyethylene (HDPE), 44
Higman, M. A., 121n60
histamine reaction, 12, 17, 49
history of DMSO, 4–8
   ban, 6
   thalidomide drug disaster, 6
holistic healing, 17
Homeopathic Treatment of Small Animals, The, 106
Houwing, Ronald, 18nn36, 37
Huang, Z., 119n38
Humble, Jim, 47
hydrotherapy, 73
hypoxia, 29

I

infections, 105
infusions, 87
injuries, 64, 105
intravenous DMSO, 79
ischemic stroke, 29

J

Jacob, Stanley W., 4–5, 66, 116nn5, 6, 8, 118n28, 119nn41, 43, 47, 122nn81, 82
Jayaveera, K. N., 124n101
Johnson, M., 118n29
Joneja, Janice, 49
juvenile rheumatoid arthritis (JRA), 70

K

Kalcker, Andreas, 47
Kaneda, T., 120n52
Kaplan, R. S., 119n42, 120n49
Kashino, Genro, 119n44
Kleberger, K. E., 123n89
Kovacs, I. B., 118nn27, n31
Kovak, W., 118n26
Kratochvílová, Irena, 116n1

L

Lackey, Homer B., 117n15
Leake, Chauncey D., 116n3
Leger, Tony, St., 123n93
Levy, Juliette de Baïracli, 106
Lexchin, Joel, 123n94
life-threatening effect, 49
Light, Donald W., 123n94
liniment, 87
Liu, Yong, 119n44
Lockwood, B., 124n107
low-density polyethylene (LDPE), 44
Luo, Y., 119n38
lupus arthritis, 70
Luza, Segisfredo, 123nn87, 88

M

MacLeod, George, 106
magnesium, 59–60

bursitis, 61–62
carpal tunnel syndrome, 62–63
cavities, 72
chronic bursitis, 61
cold sores, 77–78
DMSO concentrations chart,
  54–55
ears, 73–74
eye health, 68–70
first aid and wounds, 78
frozen shoulder, 63
hair growth, 75
head trauma, 66–67
headaches, 59–60
hemorrhoids, 76–77
injuries, 64
intravenous DMSO, 79
juvenile rheumatoid arthritis
  (JRA), 70
lupus arthritis, 70
mental health, 67–68
migraines, 59–60
muscle repair, 73
ocular migraines, 59
osteoarthritis (OA), 60–61, 70
pain-relieving, 60
pains, 56–57
persistent shingles, 77–78
restless leg syndrome (RLS), 71
rheumatoid arthritis (RA), 70
second-degree burns, 58
sinuses, 74
skin care, 75–76
tendinitis, 65–66
third-degree burns, 58

V
vasodilation increase, 29–30
Vein Tonic, 56

Veterinary Materia Medica, A, 106
Viadur, 110
Vickery, Alison, 121n70
vitamin B6, 62
vitamin B12, 62–63
vitamin C, 62, 63, 69, 89–91
vitamin D, 61
vitamin K2, 61

W
water-soluble molecules, 9
Weiser, P. B., 118n30
Weissmann, G., 118n32
Whitaker, Julian, 18
Whitesides, George M., 121n66
Wilkins, D. J., 117n17
Wolff, J., 121n63
wounds, 30, 78
wound spray, 99–100
Wright, Jonathan, 62
Wu, Y., 119n38

Y
Yamashita, K., 120n56

Z
Zeiger, M., 118n30

Acknowledgments

Writing a book is harder than I thought and more rewarding than I could have ever imagined. There were some late nights and early mornings and times when I really had to push myself beyond what I thought I was capable of.

My family looked out for me. My parents helped me to get a contractor for the new floors and even took my elderly dog to their home, which opened up more time and reduced my stress. Grandpa Gerry helped to take care of my daughter so I could get some focused time. I am grateful to my family for these acts of affection, they were truly vital.

Being a single mother and entrepreneur, the book-writing process took away the time I would normally use for social activities and seeing friends. My life became very isolated, and many connections dropped away. I did a lot of reading and researching for this book, which takes focused, quiet, thoughtful time. And there was no remaining time or energy for socializing, especially while keeping up with a thriving business!

I happen to have a daughter who constantly sings. While this is lovely, when you want quiet time and you are homeschooling, it is very challenging to find! This is why I woke up early in the morning, or stayed up late into the night to write. There were days I didn't have enough patience, and I am grateful to Anwyn, my darling daughter, for understanding and for being compassionate through this process. She is proud of me and told me this many times. Thank you, Anwyn, mommy is very proud of you too!

To my sweetest friend Janene Greer, who sent me messages of encouragement and showed excitement for me when I didn't have the energy: Thank you so much, you are a pure heart and a caring friend, and your emotional support helped me more than you know.

To talented health coach Ted Hanik, who always offered me help and support, even though he is a busy father and husband, and who consistently checked in on me to see how things were going: Thank you, you are an inspiration with a heart of gold.

To Adrian Anderson, with whom I share common interests, like the crypto-market and investing, who always brought me something fun, like local spring water or new technology: Thank you, Adrian, for being there if I ever needed to talk. Just knowing that option was there for me was enough.

I couldn't have written this book without my helpful staff, Jennifer and Debra, a vital team to keep Yummy Mummy Emporium & Apothecary running smoothly. Thank you for encouraging me and for being a strong and helpful women tribe!

Thank you so much to my publishing company, Ulysses Press. When they approached me with this project I felt instantly that it was the right group of people to work with, as they support excellent writers and important works of knowledge. Thank you for trusting me with this book and for being flexible with due dates; the artist and intuitive sides of me always needs more flow and ease of process.

And thank you, dear reader, for picking up such a book to even consider reading. Whether you or a loved one have a health concern, you are a healer and want to learn more about how to help your patients, or you are simply curious about DMSO, I appreciate you, as this is knowledge that can save lives. The more who know, the more it can help.

About the Author

Amandha Dawn Vollmer holds a bachelor of science in agricultural biotechnology from the University of Lethbridge (2000) in Alberta, Canada. She has experience as a certified lab animal technician at the University of Alberta and was trained in applied kinesiology, intravenous (IV) therapy, and Reiki. Most of her life she has taken an interest in caring for the health and well-being of animals, humans, and our Earth. Her love of botanical medicine started her self-educating on the topic many years before beginning her formal medical training. She has studied homeopathy on multiple trips to India and via distance education through the British Institute of Homeopathy.

Amandha's deep research began in 2017, when she realized its powerful physical effects from her own use. This became an impassioned focus, akin to a PhD process, reading any and every book, article, and paper on the topic.

Aside from passionate learning, Amandha has a gift for designing and creating natural medicine and body care products. She is an entrepreneur and started YumNaturals Emporium Inc. in 2012 after the birth of her daughter. She collects wild plants, creates DMSO blended formulas, and enjoys making lotions, medicinal salves, and artisanal soap. She resides in Ontario, Canada. Her website is yumnaturals.com.